THE LUST FOR
MEDICAL
BEAUTY

*Life, Perseverance,
and the Pursuit of Beauty*

By Carl L. Clarke, M.H.S., RPAC

Edited by: Linda Hinkle

Published by: GWN Publishing
www.GWNPublishing.com

Cover Design: Carl L. Clarke M.H.S., RPAC

ISBN: 978-1-959608-53-0

DEDICATION

To you, my dearest reader, thank you for choosing to embark upon this literary journey. I can only hope that you travel with me while reading with an open and curious mind. I dedicate this book, "The Lust for Medical Beauty," with utmost appreciation and admiration to you.

I also dedicate this book to my most profound inspiration, my rock, and my biggest fan: my wife and best friend, Carolina. It is with absolute love and appreciation for your commitment that I offer my heartfelt thanks and gratitude.

PREFACE

Through the depths of my professional experience, research, and reflections, I was challenged to unearth the tangled tapestry of society's lust for medical beauty. I hope to challenge your worldview of beauty and its meaning including the norms that we hold dear. From the early need for physical perfection to the exploration of unconventional forms of psychological beauty healing, this book encompasses the delicate intricacies of our human yearnings.

I bestow in my humble difference to each of you a collection of my thoughts and reasoning for the promotion of you and your cherished beauty, for it is by unyielding support and empathy that gives purpose to these words and brings vitality to the ideas conveyed within them.

We live in a world where it is easy to deny the importance of facial beauty and the gravity of attractiveness as a benefit in our personal and professional lives. It is also easy to look the other way when an attractive person is offered more of anything, in part, due solely to their beauty since we are guilty of partaking in this very behavior as well. Beauty is rewarded and this act of rewarding is accepted universally as an unwritten law of mankind; it is genetically sewn into the fabric of our lives.

Beauty in essence captivates our desires but is it taught or is the recognition of beauty passed on like an instinct of the fear of fire? Whether we like to admit it or not, our longing for attractiveness has evolved into a powerful impetus, pushing the boundaries of self-improvement. This drive, deeply ingrained within us, has a rich and intriguing history that intertwines with the evolution of medicine and the desire to control our visual aging.

Exploring the enthralling origins and advancements of my career path and medical beauty as a catalyst for a revolutionary change in how we view ourselves as human beings, this book navigates through time, shedding light on our fascinating journey of aesthetic enhancement. Within these pages, we delve into the sub-specialty of medical aesthetics, unraveling the secrets of obtaining the best treatment for your beauty concerns. Together, let us embark on a captivating exploration of the endless possibilities that lie within the realm of medical beauty.

Every major company uses the beauty of a human's face to introduce its brand, products, and services to the world. From the attractiveness of the teeth to the shape of the brows is required for all aspects of business development and growth due to our inherent nature of longing for and rewarding beauty anyway it comes.

If this is in doubt, then I would challenge you to neglect your beauty regimen (make-up, hairstyles, fashionable clothing choices, etc.) for a few months and evaluate the interpersonal interactions positive vs negative at the end of this time period.

Some people are born with natural attractiveness, however, beauty is attainable for everyone and is a choice for those who dare to push the limits. The following is how I dared to 'push the limits' in my journey to ensure my clients can attain the look they wish in the world of Medical Beauty.

May this journey captivate your hearts and intrigue your minds as it has mine, and forever remind us of the power and strength we hold as humans within our unique, imperfect, and awe-inspiring beauty.

TABLE OF CONTENTS

THE LUST FOR MEDICAL BEAUTY

CHAPTER ONE

ENIGMATIC ORIGINS

Beauty and Aesthetics Unfolded

I unknowingly learned about the art of beauty while growing up in Barbados, known for its crystal clear waters, white sand beaches, and vibrant culture. Island life has pros and cons, but it was a rewarding and adventurous experience for a young impressionable lad like myself. This is where my sense of beauty began and as amazing as this may sound, even paradise has its suffering. Little did I know that the pain awaiting me would also shape my empathetic nature along with a unique perception of human beauty from the humble beginnings of a tiny island in the Caribbean.

A Journey into the Visionary Taste of this Island

Barbados is known for its beautiful beaches, rich history, and friendly locals. The island is a small, tropical paradise that offers visitors an unforgettable experience. As a Barbadian native, I can attest that this island is one of the most beautiful places in the world for a brief reality relief. There are over 75 pristine beaches, each with its unique features from roadside beaches sprinkled with overhanging coconut leaves and vibrant palm trees to outstretched picturesque green and sandy landscaped beaches lined with breeze-swaying pine trees draping its blue skies.

On the west side of the island, the beaches are calm, and the waters are tranquil especially when laid under the evening's outstretched sunsets. Visitors can enjoy the shade of coconut, palm, or almond trees that reach out over the water in a canopy style allowing you to dip your feet in the warm waters just seconds from exiting your car. The sandy beaches vary from a fine textured pale pink and bleached white to a grittier coral-like emulsion of different particle stone and shell sizes, making each beach in Barbados a unique spectacle of vibrance and art intertwined.

Moving towards the northern interior of the island by car, the scenery becomes different with every mile passed having more open space and sugarcane plantations averaging 10,000 acres among the rolling hills. The steady fields of sugarcane crops are a beautiful sight to behold just before harvest season when the crispy air is filled with the taste and aroma of molasses and sweet sugarcane juice. It's easy to feel small when standing at the top of these hills, looking out at the endless sheets of waving green against the curtain-like backdrop of the deep blue ocean that seems to engulf the island.

Heading east, the overwhelming Atlantic ocean meets the island silhouette with its endless imposition of waves creating a different style of beach experience. This is where the famous Bathsheba Beach is located. Surfing competitions are a staple for the summer/rainy/hurricane seasons with the biggest names in surfing joining in to catch some of the most ravaging waves and wicked waters. This is not an option for the novice surfer, the waves are too high, and the ocean is too rough, making it an ideal spot only for experienced surfers. However, visitors can still sit and have a picnic while enjoying the scenery and sounds of ocean breaths.

On the north side of the island, the scenery becomes more artistically intense. Some cliffs drop over hundreds of feet dramatically into the Atlantic Ocean. There are no beaches on this side of the island, and the waves can be quite frightening. However, there are openings and tunnels in the rocks that visitors can climb through to get to the ocean, and some openings that seem to go nowhere. The tunnels were likely created by slaves or captured escapees in the times of sea piracy, as they are the only way to get to the waters in some places. Beautiful Barbados has a remarkable and dangerous past that has cultivated its people of all types and backgrounds.

The landscapes of Barbados are unique and diverse and full of beauty from every angle. You just have to look. As a native, I have seen these landscapes change over the years, becoming even more captivating and diverse. The island is truly a paradise for nature lovers, and its natural beauty is one of the reasons why Barbados is such a popular tourist destination. If you ever have the chance to visit Barbados, make sure you take the time to explore the island's intriguing landscapes. You won't be disappointed.

The Beauty of Life in the Islands

Life in Barbados was full of opportunities to explore, learn, and create. Whether it was listening to the stories of the older generation conversing non-stop, exploring the island's natural beauty, or creating our own entertainment with whatever was around at the time; this included making our own toys, kites, or go carts, there was always something to make or something to do. As a child, my siblings and I were not exposed to exuberant celebrations for the holidays, birthdays or Christmas, therefore, we improvised and learned how to make something out of seemingly nothing.

At times, a simple toy or homemade Barbadian cake provided a meaningful, pleasurable, and extraordinary day. As a culture, we always kept things simple; that's island life in a nutshell. As I grew older, I discovered the joy of woodworking and metalworking, crafting and creating chairs, vases, statues, and more. I was amazed at the infinite possibilities of shaping metal and wood into what were considered beautiful objects, and for me, creating things with my hands was an absolute marvel, a gift, and it came to me as naturally as breathing. I found out very early in life that I was good with my hands, and I was the only sibling to have acquired this talent.

Nothing and nowhere is perfect and life on the island, though beautiful, also has its challenges. Growing up with a single parent and five siblings meant that there were often financial struggles although I would admit we did not grow up poor at all, quite the contrary, life was good. I knew that money was important, but it was never a goal to accumulate things. We just did not talk about money besides what our business required. Money was always only a tool to help achieve immediate and short-term goals and to help guide others such as friends and family. However, this early view of money has created challenges for me as I grew into adulthood, as I still am not comfortable negotiating or discussing money with my clients to this day.

Career Planning in a Land of Beauty

Career decisions can shape the rest of our lives and the way we live our lives by determining the jobs and opportunities that we will encounter. It is a crucial time for young students on the island when they reach the middle years of high school, and they must choose the career curriculum that will guide them toward their future successes or failures, a roulette of sorts. In retrospect, this decision should never be taken lightly or left in the hands of teenage boys and girls, but unfortunately, this was the case for me. If you choose to live on the island, it will be the only career you will likely only have as the island is genuinely small and lacks career growth or diversity. Unlike the larger countries where students make their career choices well into young adulthood, beyond 20 years old at times; in Barbados, this choice is made around 14-15 years of age, well before the age of consent, legal alcohol consumption, or the ability to drive a car. I was just not mature enough for such a colossal decision as you will come to see.

Strategic Positioning Between Bad Influences

For me, it was no different. I was approximately 14 years old when I was thrust into this dilemma to choose a permanent career path. I completed the first half of secondary high school with a customary high-grade score, now it was preparation for the second phase where the general curriculum would change to career-shaping studies. I was uncertain about what I wanted to do. I chose a path that combined my interests in building and the arts, which led me to an engineering curriculum, which made sense, so why was I in a sewing and needle-work class?

It all started with what I believed to be a casual decision. I had to choose which classes I would take for my career studies and was faced with a difficult choice between the classes that my best friend was taking and the classes that would lead me to my true calling. At 14 years of age, an adolescent is not mentally equipped to make or handle such a profound decision, and ultimately, in my juvenile mind, I did not want to give up the joys of a perfect union with my best friend and our shenanigans.

I inevitably followed the fun and succumbed to his influence on me thereby choosing the classes he would be taking. Unfortunately, it led to a more uncertain future for me but revealed a dichotomy of two personalities in me: a classic scenario for my birth sign Gemini. It was one of the worst decisions I had ever made, choosing my future based on another person's interests. These actions taught me valuable and profound lessons about life, friendships, and decision-making.

Social Status: Opportunity and Resources

There were two types of students in high school, the upper-class students and the lower-class students. The upper class were the elitist students who enjoyed a certain privilege geared toward becoming top socialites. The elitists often but not always, got higher grades in sciences, math, social studies, and other demanding aristocratic studies. The lower-class, on the other hand, were the students who struggled with their studies, their emotions, and their ability to follow the protocols and rules levied against them. Classes such as needlework and introductory typing were interlaced with sports and recreational activities. They were seemingly being led to a world of subjugation and control.

Unfortunately, my best friend was part of the latter, and I was part of the former exposed to the latter but confident in my aptitude with an insanely high self-esteem, confidence, and pride. Although my grades were A's and some occasional B's, I wanted to stay with my best friend and by default, the lower class, the connections and loyalty meant a lot to me then. So, I followed him and his choices into the lower-class group. You see, the entertainment value I received prevented me from being bored in class. I was never one to stand still and quietly work. Looking back then, I would definitely diagnose my younger self as a clear and classic case of Attention Deficit Hyperactivity Disorder. I was a dreamer, an independent thinker, and later, a loner.

My poor decision-making led to many problems and numerous regrets, but it also made me into a stronger, empathetic individual seeing the world from multiple perspectives at a young age. I guess I was fortunate?! The conversations and attitudes of these two groups were vastly different. The elite group talked about work, politics, world affairs, economics, and other serious topics guided by their studies and interspersed with the normal teenage hyperbole and exaggerations about teenage life surrounding girls and possessions.

The lower-class group were excited more about confrontations, sexual encounters, and other trivial matters due to a lack of care, interest, or know-how from their educators, a similar situation we see in urban cities that would build low-income project housing and abandon their residents without the resources to thrive. This is what I witnessed at an early age. Now, there was certainly an overlap in the behaviors of these two groups but the typical everyday conversation of the two groups mirrored the homes of the students and reflected what was thought by the people of influence in their lives. The lower-class's words and actions reflected the sentiment and education of their households begging the question whether the lives of many are due to nature versus nurture.

When I was engaged with the upper-class group, everything was fine, I was fine, and still in the top three to five of the class grades, but when I was with the lower-class group, though I blended in and was also fine, I still felt a sense of embarrassment and feeling out of place among them. Within the lower-class group, however, there was never a dull moment. My teachers and upper-class friends wondered why I was there with this group, to the point of openly asking how I ended up with the lower classes, and it was in these times when I truly felt like I didn't belong to either group. Neither warranted my affiliation.

I vividly remembered having a conversation in school on the center field lawn of the volleyball court with one of my upper-class friends and remembering his hatred of the lower-class group and me explaining that I need to be there to have more classes in metal, wood, and tailoring shop and had to be with them to fulfill these credits. This was obviously a lie and a feeble attempt, at best, to hide the fact that I decided to join their classes because of my loyalty to my friend in the lower-class group. This would have sounded stupid and would have painted me as the dummy I felt I was each and every day. I know I was stuck between both worlds with no possibility of escaping the condescending looks of the upper-class group and the embarrassment of being seen with the lower-class group. To make matters worse, my friendship with my best friend was gradually weakening as I matured and my interests widened. I was shedding my childhood naivete and realizing my place among my peers and the real world.

As time took its toll, seemingly causing damage to my previous playful and innocent soul, I realized that I had indeed made a terrible mistake. I had let my loyalty to my friend cloud my judgment and I had chosen the wrong path for my career studies. However, at that age, was it truly loyalty to my friend or loyalty to the fun I had with him? I should have taken the path that was right for me, not the one that my friend had chosen that was right for him. I began to regret my decision and wished I had chosen differently. I was awake. I still remember feeling the sharp blade of regret cutting into my prospects from this poor decision. To this day, that experience continues to shape my connections and my judgments in my older and wiser age.

Thankfully, Shakespeare's famous quote "All's well that ends well" (credited to but not his original work) was certainly reflected upon me. In the end, I learned some valuable lessons from my experiences. First, I learned that friendship should not come before major or potential life-changing decisions, it will remain if the friendship is true.

Second, you must choose the path that is right for you, even if it means hurting others by parting ways with your friends. True friends will remain friends even if miles apart.

Third, I learned that every decision has consequences, good and bad, and you must be prepared to live with the consequences. If you make the wrong choice, you must face the consequences, learn from it, and make it well in the end. Yes, all decisions can be made positively depending on how you perceive it or change your perspective about the way you view the problem and handle it.

Fourth, I learned that there is no shame in being part of a lower-class group. Many are born into less favorable groups with a seemingly impossible way to overcome them. It doesn't define who you are, and it doesn't mean that you're not smart or capable. It just means that our paths in life are set very differently with challenges that can make or break us regardless of our status, wealth, or social standing in life, which makes us unique and our distinctive paths exclusive.

Prelude to Peril: Safety Before Beauty

As students, we are always reminded of the safety measures when operating machinery, especially when it comes to iron welding and using heavy machinery for cutting wood. One of those measures was using safety helmets with a heavily tinted window visor to protect our eyes from the high arc of the welding torches. However, one day, I experienced another life-changing moment while operating the arc welder in my metal shop class.

I found it cumbersome to keep moving my helmeted goggles on and off my head to get the correct placement of my welding rods. In a moment of carelessness and a lack of appreciation for the dangers that always abound, I gave myself an few extra seconds to glimpse at the arc without my protective helmet. What a glorious sight to behold—the intensity of the arc light was unlike no other sight—leaving an imprinted glowing halo of green, blue, and orange that remained for several minutes. This occurred several times that morning without consequence. I also had a very normal day of classes and socializing, but at the end of the school day, I found that I was unable to open my eyes without intense pain due to an unusual feeling of grit or sand in my eyes.

This is one of the most irritating and painful feelings you can endure, and we all know what it feels like to have a particle of dust fly into our eye, now add soap for the burning sensation and increase the particle size several times. This feeling culminated into a sandy, gritty, and severe pain along with an intense burn that rendered me 100 percent blind. There was nothing but complete darkness and I had a fear of opening my eyes.

Completely bewildered, I was the last one to leave the school because of the embarrassment I felt at my self-imposed problem. The task at hand now was how to get home before it got dark. I could not just call for help, there were no cell phones then. I had to navigate a one-mile path home, step by step, with my eyes closed 100% of the time. This was a scary and humbling moment for me since one of the neighborhoods I had to traverse was not overly welcoming but I am sure everyone knew something was wrong with me as I hugged the sides of walls and plants while shuffling forward.

First, I was incapable of seeing anyone to ask for help, and second, my navigation was accomplished by remembering the terrain, touching the trees, shrubs, stone walls, and galvanized sheet metal house siding that lined the hilly and rocky terrain all the way to my home. One slow step at a time, now I could just imagine what people must have thought as they saw me struggling along the way at a snail's pace.

At last, I had never been so elated to arrive home. I remember touching the leaves of the shrubs and the hedges lining my house and feeling the walls to the permanently open gate and finally the side of the house before I was at ease knowing I was safely home. I took 15 steps toward the front door with my arms outstretched until I touched the doorknob, then opened the door and another 20 steps navigating inside the house while touching the side of the living room and kitchen walls on my way to my bedroom door. I then climbed into my bed quietly avoiding anyone who may have arrived at home. I did not tell my mother for fear of being punished, and I truly believed I was blind and would never see again.

So, like any reserved, introspective normal teenager, I decided to wait out my blindness, contemplate in my mind all the horrors of being blind and see what happened the next day. Fingers crossed! I surprisingly slept very well that night considering the harrowing experience I endured. Upon opening my eyes slowly, after taking a moment to touch them to confirm they were still there and noticing that the excruciating pain had subsided, I was able to faintly see first the bedroom ceiling with some discomfort, but nothing like I had experienced several hours prior. In retrospect, I evidently had suffered a high-arc injury: excessive ultraviolet radiation and ionizing damage to my eyes that caused severe swelling and irritation to the corneas, preventing me from opening my eyes, causing temporary blindness, and excruciating pain and headaches with debilitating light sensitivity.

This experience typically lasts a little under 24 hours and, if continued, can lead to permanent disabilities. I was lucky. After this experience, I went on to do exceptionally well in my metalworking classes with a new appreciation for safety measures and protocols. I was still driven to finish my projects and make the most beautiful objects I could with the class curriculum and supplies given. It was my passion for art and creative studies that motivated me to continue after such a formidable experience.

In conclusion, the experience taught me a valuable lesson about the importance of safety measures when using any tool or mechanical device. It only takes one brief moment of carelessness to change your entire life forever. I hope that my experience serves as a reminder to everyone to take safety measures seriously towards yourself and others and to not take risks with your health and well-being.

Taking a step further into my journey, one year had passed, and my classes were more tailored and directed toward the culmination of the previous years and my chosen career path. I was more involved now in architectural, mechanical, and engineering drawing. Understanding geometry, mathematics, line theory, and building theory, and being able to orient around schematics of buildings, machine parts, or any mechanical device was a new experience for me. To that point, my goal while living in Barbados was to become a mechanical engineer and I was accepted to one of the best engineering schools to commence after my high school graduation. There seem to be always twists and turns along this journey, however, my graduation did not happen, and so too, my first day in mechanical engineering school did not come to pass.

Sinister Transformations: Beauty Emerges Out of Suffering

The beginning of my realization that I wanted to alleviate suffering as part of my profession came from an incident that happened when I was quite young. While we know that suffering is a part of life, and it builds character and shapes who we become as adults, an empathetic person witnessing someone else's suffering can be overwhelming, especially when you're powerless to help them (and the size of a small twig).

A friend of my mother at the time was a bosomy, full-figured, young woman, with long reddish hair and a heavenly face. For a 10-year-old boy, remembering her looks as vividly as if it were yesterday, she must have been a very beautiful woman. She often wore bright red lipstick that gave her face a particularly striking and seductive appearance. My mother would often ask me to check on her or to just deliver messages and so I would eagerly walk the few blocks to her house, ready to please.

One day, upon my arrival and after knocking on the door for what seemed to be an eternity, she opened the door, and everything changed for me that day. I found Shelley-ann as I had never seen her before, collapsing on the floor and sobbing uncontrollably. I had never seen anyone look so defeated and broken before. My mother was not a crier, and I had never seen her, or any woman close to me cry. In West Indian life, unlike the U.S., women or men don't cry. So, to my startling surprise, I didn't know what to do or to say. All I could do was watch as she cried, feeling helpless and useless in my cut-off jeans and flip-flops. I do remember saying, "Umm, my mother gave me this parcel for you to have." I was completely out of my comfort zone, and this is where I believe my empathetic nature started to awaken.

Looking back, I realize that Shelley-ann was the victim of psychological and physical abuse, and it wasn't her fault. But at the time, I didn't understand any of that. My world was playing, laughing, seeking new pleasures, and avoiding responsibility just like any other kid my age. At that moment, all I knew was that I wanted to take away her pain and make her feel better. This experience has stayed with me throughout my entire life, always reminding me of my wish to unburden pain.

It was encounters such as these that guided me towards my present life's purpose and ultimately to the position where I find the greatest comfort. As the connection between my clients and myself develop, their personal growth and healing also evolve, along with the treatment and conversational boundaries. I receive two distinct types of patients: those seeking solely beautification treatments and those seeking inner healing. This process takes time to unfold, and it is the patient and empathetic practitioner who will reap the most rewards and provide the most benefits.

Empathy: The Vital Ingredient in Aesthetic Medicine

As I sit here writing this chapter, I can't help but reflect on the significant impact being an empath has had on my life. It's funny to think that the word "empath" wasn't even a part of my vernacular until a few years ago when I was talking with one of my employees, now a close friend, who also happens to be an empath. She explained to me why we were alike and introduced me to a whole new understanding of my own experiences and purpose among others. Empaths are individuals with a heightened awareness of their surroundings and an intuition of the feelings of others in their immediate vicinity.

Being an empath means that I am highly attuned to the emotions of those around me. There are different types of empaths, but for me, it mainly falls into a combination of cognitive + intuitive empathy. This means that I have the ability to understand where another person's frame of reference is coming from and to see through the emotional barriers that they may have erected to protect themselves.

Another aspect of being an empath is the ability to sense another person's intentions. This is where reading body language and voice inflections come into play. It's amazing how much you can learn about someone just by listening to them and observing their behavior.

There is the emotional empath, which is the ability to feel another person's pain, suffering, and joy. While I have less of this ability, I still find it incredibly powerful to be able to understand and truly feel the emotions of those around me without becoming too emotionally invested in myself. This allows me to separate my patient's psychological and physical pain from my personal life.

Empath practitioners have double the tasks in treating their patients; there is an emotional toll the body endures and if we do not take care to heal, we will implode upon ourselves and lash out by being defiant and antagonistic to push the sensory overload away. We are misunderstood at times, and we must defend our own psychological health.

The positive expression of the golden rule of empathy is to treat others as you would like to be treated. While this is a noble goal, it's important to remember that everyone has different needs and preferences. This is where understanding your audience is the real game-changer that comes into play. By being attuned to the emotions of those around you, you can better understand what they need and how to best help them.

When a client sits in my treatment chair, everything around me halts. I instantly forget my own emotions and I am entirely theirs for the duration of the treatment visit. In the end, being an empath has been both a blessing and a curse. It can be overwhelming at times, but it has also allowed me to connect with others in ways that no other can, on a deeper level, and to help alleviate their suffering. We empaths should all be grateful for this gift and strive to use it to make a positive impact in the world.

I was fortunate to be surrounded by Barbados's natural beauty which left an indelible mark on my soul. The azure waters, pristine beaches, and vibrant flora nurtured my appreciation for beauty in all its forms. Little did I know that this appreciation would set the stage for a new chapter in my life, leading me down a path that combines my love for beauty, the virtue of empathy, and the attributes of engineering.

THE LUST FOR MEDICAL BEAUTY

CHAPTER TWO

EMBRACING THE UNKNOWN

Leaving the Past and Anticipating the Unforeseen

Death of the inner child occurs for our rebirth into adulthood, and this is met with much conflict and turmoil within ourselves directed toward our caretakers because of a lack of understanding: time to leave the nest. As adulthood approached, the feeling of not belonging, not being in a place where I could grow and flourish was becoming ever more evident and ever more real. I somehow was no longer at home in my paradise as I no longer loved my environment. To this day, one of my famous quotes is "You can't live in paradise; you can visit but you cannot stay." For me, Barbados had become my paradise but no longer my home. Where do I belong? The mounting anxiety about being anywhere in the world other than Barbados grew over the passing months. Death was becoming.

It was in 1989 that I landed on American soil for the first time, and I couldn't help but feel an emotional mix of excitement and anxiety. I had always been intrigued by the United States, and I had finally had the chance to take a summer vacation here. I was elated when I was chosen out of my siblings to go to the United States, possibly on vacation or longer. I understood why I was the one chosen, not because I was special but because I was different. I was asked and I accepted the offer wholeheartedly. I had an interesting perspective on people and my surroundings and saw things somewhat differently.

However, I also knew that this trip could potentially change my life forever. If I fell in love with the country, there was an opportunity for me to stay and pursue my education there. I accepted the invitation to leave Barbados with what seemed to be my mother's lifetime stockpile of US $2 bills totaling a whopping $200 and that was just fine with me. Nothing says adventure more than a duffle bag of clothes and a King James Bible stuffed with $2 bills!

My expectations of the United States were grandiose, to say the least. I, like many other West Indian children and adults, viewed the annual JCPenney catalog as the Bible to the world of the United States and its fortunes. It seemed like everything you could ever want, or need, and was beautifully laid out with exceptional graphics of just about everything you could ever wish for. The marketing tactics in the JCPenney catalog, as I see now, made you embrace the United States as the superior continent with everything you want arriving at your doorstep at a moment's notice. Marketing is a bitch but so necessary for fortunes to be made. Marketing is cunning, conniving, captivating, and enticing, however, never 100% truthful and seldom trustworthy.

My initial impressions of the U.S. were based on what I had seen on the big screen and on television. I imagined grand cities filled with towering skyscrapers and bustling streets, and friendly people who were always eager to help a stranger. However, the reality that I encountered was quite different. Upon landing at JFK International Airport in Queens, NY, my expectations of the United States were innocent at best, however, that innocence was fleeting. I was 17 and unlike 17-year-olds in this country, my mind was not forced to mature rapidly from a pivotal point of survival, but now, this new environment meant I, too, had to focus on survival.

The very evening I landed in early July was dark, overcast with some intermittent showers, and I remember being packed into a compact-sized car for five being driven for what felt like hours through the streets of Brooklyn. As we drove west on the Eastern Parkway, I saw what resembled a war zone of toppled and vacant buildings all covered in graffiti and littered with homeless victims lining the sidewalk and lurking along the alleyways. This was my first hour in the United States; it was a stark contrast to that JCPenney catalog. I clutched my duffle bag closer in my lap and waited.

What happened to the picturesque cityscapes with tranquil neighborhoods, the clean streets with nothing but the latest model cars carrying the perfect families around town? I had left the homelessness-free Barbados I had grown up in and now as exasperated as I may have been, something still compelled me to widen my eyes, take a deep breath, clutch my duffel bag and bible again, and get comfortable because this was it: this was my new home.

By no choice of my own, I quickly adapted to my new surroundings. I learned the street vernacular, donned the dress code, and always looked over my shoulders. I realized that life in the United States was not what I had imagined and that it was up to me to make the most of it. I worked hard, made connections, and did whatever I had to have a life of my choosing. For most of us, life is filled with perils of varying degrees, and nothing gets better unless you actively work toward making it so. For maximum benefit, you must lead the change or be led by the change, your choice.

Looking back thus far, I realize that my expectations of the United States were unrealistic, but hey, I was only 17 and it didn't mean that the United States wasn't the land of opportunity. The United States is neither good nor bad, it is a business entity, it just is created for maximum profit by its creators. Our perceptions and actions give us the world we live in, there is no such thing as Mother Nature, these are romanticized terms we offer up to make sense of the world we live in and the circumstances out of our control. This world will eat you up if you make too many mistakes rich or poor. It just means that sometimes, the reality of life doesn't match up with our expectations unless we make it so. It's up to us to adapt, persevere, and make the most of the opportunities presented to us especially if we view every circumstance as a potential opportunity, good or bad. And to that, I was just getting started.

A Sub-human Life: Paying the Price for the Adventure and Appreciating the Cost

It's a bewildering experience to exist in a foreign land without being seen, representing the stateless souls. Invisibility has its pros but not when you want to be seen, heard, loved. Life in the U.S. is incredibly difficult and demoralizing if you are between adequate resident documentation. Barbados has experienced its share of immigrants from other West Indian islands. We all must understand that migration is a normal act all around the world based on the life created by elected officials from tribesmen to presidents/prime ministers, and kings and queens. Many migrants are forced to leave their country, while others negate the risk and choose the adventure and potential victories ahead. This is how America was built. I left not because of poverty; I chose to leave from a sense of adventure and growth.

I had hoped to complete two years of high school and start college majoring in architecture or engineering, but without official immigration papers, which were not ready at the time, and seemingly delayed, that dream quickly collapsed. As someone who had always championed the underdog, I found myself being the under-underdog and fighting to survive. But it was not over yet!

Journey of Discovery: Finding Beauty Without a Map

Now, at this pivotal moment, I was 18 years old, and there was no parental figure I could turn to for an allowance to buy the simple daily needs for my teenage life, so I ventured into my first cosmetic/beauty gig. I had become a street barber charging $8 a haircut and $10-$12 for a cut with designs. I was finally able to buy my first Asics Gel sneakers and designer sweatpants, one red pair and one blue pair. I was no longer shackled to an impoverished look in the U.S. which made me more appealing to all and popular among many, but also reduced my risk of being attacked in the streets, pulled over by the police, or threatened while in my heavily protected Jewish neighborhood of Crown Heights.

The word "street" preceding a noun to describe a job screams of dangerous on-gongs, and at times, I was cutting hair way past midnight, using the dim light cast of the streetlamps to highlight the skulls of my patrons and deliver a breathtaking work of art. It is quite likely that everyone whose hair I was cutting had a gun on them. The street language in the hood was different, you had to survive, and every turn was an inconvenient truth waiting to take you down: the cops, the neighborhood gangs, the government system in place to box you in, and just about anyone who was not your relative or friend. Working for cash in the streets as a barber was not necessarily free of conflict or crime, if you asked me how I circumvented this jungle of hatred and deceit, I cannot tell you how in so many words, I just did!

However, I can say, when you are determined to survive and have the necessary intellectual skills - street and otherwise - you will find a way. The work was hard and dangerous, to say the least, but it was my only option. It was during this time that I truly understood the harsh realities of the average life in America. When you don't have the proper documentation or the right connections, it can feel like the world is against you. You are stateless, unrepresented, and invisible.

Despite the challenges, giving up is not a variable in the equation for success. Without laboring on the thoughts of the low prospects around me, staying focused and fighting to achieve seemed to be a built-in feature, I was somehow hardwired to power through adversity. After two long years of waiting, I was able to obtain a proper, legitimate immigration status but first, I had to go back to Barbados to get everything in order before I was able to re-enter the United States with a green card. I was no longer sub-human, I was a human again, still me, and now even more driven.

As I settled into my new life, I couldn't help but notice the stark contrast between the life I had left behind in Barbados and the one I was now living. Crime and drug-afflicted souls and victims of the era's circumstances painted the streets and alleyways making it a normal sight to behold. This was just another day in the land of opportunity. It was hard to believe that my mother and siblings were living a better life back home in tiny Barbados with a mere 258,000 inhabitants, far less than the population of Brooklyn, NY with a whooping 1,166,582 people back then in 1990.

I knew that I had a chance to create the life I wanted despite the country's failings. My pre-legal immigration status in the U.S. had taught me that life was full of ups and downs, but it was up to me to keep pushing forward and never give up on what I believed to be mine. Shortly after this humbling experience, I stumbled upon a volunteer program for mentally challenged kids. While I knew that I didn't exactly fit the demographic they were looking for, I was eager to help in any way that I could, especially since the program was conducted in the city hospitals.

It was there that I met Mr. Paul, one of the program directors who saw potential in me and felt that he could help. The program was a city-sponsored volunteer opportunity for challenged urban kids and there were many spaces available for me to help while I continued to seek employment. Mr. Paul took me to the Cardio-Thoracic Intensive Care Unit (CT-ICU) at Maimonides Medical Center where my roots took hold and my mind opened like no other time in my life.

The potential in this hospital was massive. I was able to reach the level of floor coordinator, well, volunteer floor coordinator charged with retrieving and storing charts, organizing the notes station, and addressing visitors on the overhead P.A. system. This volunteer position was the highest level for the volunteers, but I still didn't feel like I belonged to this group, something was missing, and there had to be more.

Paying my bills meant I had to push harder and so after months of searching, I was able to procure a position as a bank teller in Park Slope Brooklyn, a very upscale and quaint neighborhood that was a far cry from my death-ridden Brooklyn lodging. This was about to change. Being a bank teller was my first job outside of the manual labor I was used to. It was paying minimum wage of $7+ an hour at the time of hire, but the responsibility was immense. I had to go through a lot of credentialing and test taking to prove I was competent enough to count money, give change, and handle large sums of cash.

The reality is that this was not foreign to me. In Barbados, I did just this every day. My mother was the owner of a typical West Indian liquor shop. We sold alcohol, groceries, and anything small enough to handle and carry by hand out of the shop. I was introduced to commerce from at 9 years old. The cursing, the drinking, the smoking, and any and everything you could hear from drunk adults well past midnight was a normal evening for me. My brothers and I often fell asleep to the occasional fights and arguments that brewed forth from as early as the afternoon on some days. This was my childhood, and I loved every part of it, mostly.

Navigating the Judicial System: A Lesson in Inequity

Mr. Paul was able, through the volunteer program, to get a free train pass for me so I could travel to and from Maimonides Medical Center every day. Though the train pass allowed me to save money, affording daily travel to volunteer and work was taking a toll on my meager earnings as a minimum wage bank teller and something just had to give.

My first legal encounter with the NYC judicial system left an impression that followed me and allowed me to further navigate the paths ahead of me. This was a normal day with nothing out of the ordinary except that I had forgotten my free train pass in my volunteer jacket at the hospital. My train from the neighborhood of the hospital that passes every 15 - 20 minutes was fast approaching the station, and the station clerk who would normally open the gates for students or individuals branding a train pass was ignoring my pleas to open the gate. Now, I know the station clerk had seen me for the past several months, and I felt that he was intentionally avoiding eye contact, which led me to do something that I have never done and never would again. I jumped the turnstile and proceeded in the direction of my train.

In my defense, my immature mind concluded that I should jump the turnstile as I do possess a train pass, it was just not on my person at the time. Well, on that day, around the corner were two NYC transit officers waiting for unsuspected turnstile jumpers, which I believe was a major problem for the NYC transit system back then. I was stopped and charged with a violation for jumping the turnstile.

I remember having a sense of frustration and disappointment at the same time. Frustration at the system for not seeing my point of view, which was valid, and disappointment at myself for making such a bad decision regardless of the circumstance. It was my first real lesson in the racial strife and minority disparities that many people still have to endure today. I was given a citation to appear in court, where I vigorously claimed my innocence, showing them my up-to-date pass and explaining the situation. But despite my evidence and clear innocence through bad decision making, I was still found guilty. Intent did not play a part in the decision to create a record for my poor deed.

I couldn't understand how this was possible, especially since I had proven that I had a valid pass and was within my allotted time frame for travel. Well, we can't win it all. The circumstance and the intent did not match the punishment. Punishment I endured by paying the fine and having a criminal record levied against me by a court arbitrator. I was lucky though; these were the lessons I needed to circumvent the judicial system regarding the treatment of individuals like me. I had to learn that although I may not be a bad person, a stranger in a uniform will only see me as black and treat me according to his/her biases.

This experience opened my eyes to the harsh reality that many minorities face in this country. Minorities seldom get a slap on the wrist. Instead, they are branded hooligans and criminals, given criminal records for further evidence/proof later in their lives if involved in any legal negative activity, small or minor, that they are indeed career criminals. We are often not given the same leeway or benefit of the doubt as others. Minorities are not allowed to make mistakes and are held to a higher standard.

What's even more frustrating is that the judge or arbitrator who oversaw my case was a black woman. It was puzzling to me that someone who looked like me could still be a part of such a negative system that so easily punishes or incarcerates people for minor offenses. I walked away from this experience being more aware of the systemic injustices that exist in our society and to always be vigilant in fighting against them. I learned my lesson and never made the mistake of jumping over a turnstile again, but the memory of that day still lingers with me. It serves as a reminder that we still have a long way to go toward achieving true equality and justice for all.

Curiosity Didn't Kill the Cat: My Three Saints

Well into the volunteer program, I witnessed three medical specialists in white coats reading x-rays on the backlight corridor wall and was just curious as to who there were since they were on my floor, and I needed to know everyone who ventured on my floor. They informed me that they were physician assistants and attending one of the patients on the floor post-cardiac surgery. I cannot state in words the excitement that came over me and that I knew this was where I was going to be. This was my new goal. My new Ah-Ha! moment. I was going to be a Physician Assistant.

Shortly after I applied to five colleges/universities, which was all I could afford at the time. And, after a few weeks, I was enrolled in St. John's University Physician Assistant Program. I would now have to somehow fit a total of six years of Bachelor of Science (four years) and the Physician Assistant Certification course (four years) into four straight years without summer vacation or winter breaks. This seemed to be the culmination of my mechanical engineering studies, being able to read and reconstruct blueprints of buildings and structures, as well as deconstruct and reconstruct mechanical parts such as engines and turbines. But how would I use this knowledge in the medical field? I guess my path seemed to be going into an entirely different path than I hoped or expected but there was no roadmap for confirmation. I would never have known these skills attained in Barbados would help me excel in all science courses culminating in a near 4.0 GPA.

As I slowly left the CT-ICU floor for the last time, I couldn't help the feeling that my life had changed irreversibly by the interactions with people who cared. I wanted to be one of those people. I wanted to touch the souls of others in need. Well, wishes and wholesome advice is what I remembered most. I loved that place. I had also left Brooklyn behind; no more evening shoot-outs, robberies, or drug sales in my building's vestibule. No more nonsense. This was truly the beginning of the rest of my life.

I was still working at the bank in Brooklyn and after a few promotions, I was almost at \$8/hour, \$7.97 per hour to be exact. I was able to afford a small room to share and bounced around from room to room approximately seven times in Queens while attending my first year at St. John's University Queens campus. Looking for single rooms to share on my meager minimum wage earnings was challenging to say the least but it taught me how to live and appreciate going without.

Some of the places I lived in were not too hospitable, and some were unquestionably unsafe, especially the basement rooms that were void of windows. Looking back on Brooklyn today gives me the acknowledgment that adversity can be overcome with discipline, hard work and having the determination to create a life you envision.

Finding a Place I Finally Belonged

Up until this point I had never sat in a luxury vehicle, but as I sat in a colleague's car who offered me a ride to school one day after seeing me at the bus stop I realized that I had chosen the right path and was reassured with a glimpse of the future to come. It was tough though, seeing my schoolmates driving BMWs and Mercedes Benz' while I was struggling to make ends meet. But I had to be laser focused and stay determined. I had the energy to do so much in so little time at such a young age, and studying was never a problem; I was still an academic sponge. I absorbed everything, I learned easily, and did great on my examinations.

I was becoming more conscious of minority struggles and the disparities among us and what bothered me more than anything else was the disregard for education many of my fellow minority students had. The countless house parties, skipping classes, and meager grades I witnessed in many American blacks, not the African blacks, or the European blacks, or the Middle-Eastern blacks, nor the Caribbean blacks, but the American Blacks. Seeing how many of the American black students acted made me question their understanding of what they were throwing away by not making education a priority.

Especially when you are the first or only child in the family to attend college and threw it away by choosing obsolete (to black students) majors not designed to propel a person to financial success but to just have another job at best. Many called these curriculum courses white majors, and many minorities fell prey to this custom of finally reaching college, graduating, and working in menial jobs. This was not me anymore, making decisions based upon other people's choices or friendships. No, I would never make that mistake again, and so I thank my high school days in Barbados when the wrong decisions were made. I learned.

The problem for me was integrating into new groups, societies, and people, seeing the disparities, and going along with it. It was something that always bothered me tremendously. I found it challenging to join groups like fraternities and be a part of something that didn't align with my values.

Fortunately, even with my tight schedule, I still found time to do some extracurricular activities on the university grounds. I was able to get on the junior-level fencing team at St. John's University but that was it, no time for any other leisure activities. I didn't have a lot of friends to hang out with, so it was mostly school from 5:30 a.m. to 1-2 p.m. and work from 4 p.m. to 9 p.m., then home by 11 p.m. if the trains ran on time.

The first-year medical school physician assistant training is by far the most difficult set of courses that I have ever undertaken. If physician assistant studies were a sport, it would be a decathlon and the M.D. study curriculum would be a marathon. Physician assistant studies is an all-around academic barrage of medical specialties all tucked into a 2-year program including 10 months of residency for all specialties combined.

The curriculum, in its design, is a momentous achievement that cannot be debated by any other area of study or by any other medical professional study. The wording of "assistant" in the title of physician assistant, now "Physician Associate" is erroneously at best and misleading by misguiding people/patients to judge the physician assistant as an assistive role or "Assistant to the Physician." Being a physician assistant is the one career where you constantly must educate and reassure your patient that you are not an assistant but a board-certified medical professional instrumental in their diagnosis, management, and care of them. Now imagine seeing 30- 40 patients per day and having this discussion that takes up 2-10 minutes of the patient visit.

Affirmation: Meeting the Challenges

I finally graduated from both St. John's University and Bayley Seton Physician Assistant Program in the same year and time with a Bachelor of Science on one hand and a Certificate to Practice Medicine on the other. This was now the beginning of what I was working toward ever since the days volunteering in the CT-ICU Maimonides

Medical Center and speaking to those three physician assistants at the X-ray booth.

Above the double doors of the famous Brooklyn Library Eastern Parkway Branch a sign reads: "A journey of a thousand miles begins with a single step." This was my new home dusk till dawn seven days a week where breakfast, lunch, and dinner were ordered and eaten. In preparation for my certification examinations, 10 medical specialties had to be studied for one six-hour examination. No pressure at all. I pushed through my board certification examinations studies and then waited for my results patiently. I remember the feeling of complete numbness after I made the last stroke of my keyboard in the examination center. I was done with studying, done with dinner wraps, done with hard library chairs, done with reciting medical study phrases, I was done! Several days later, my anxiety was quenched by the sight of a passing grade. I was now a Board Certified Physician Assistant. I had reached my goal!

Searching for Just the Right Job

I was now a Board-Certified Physician Assistant looking to make a mark and show any hospital that would have me that I was the real deal. However, another wake-up call was waiting for me; I had the real world to contend with. My need to find a meaningful job proved to be a major hurdle beyond belief. My marriage was in turmoil, my son was now two years old, and I was now 27. A new medical grad should have no problems finding a job, especially as a physician assistant, right? Well, despite my best efforts, I found myself struggling to secure at the very least, a basic interview. I scoured the newspapers, circled every PA listing I could find, and sent out more resumes than I thought possible. I pounded the pavement up and down the Manhattan streets with no luck for several months, then finally, nine months later, I had a series of alternative medicine jobs that just didn't quite cut it for me.

In the desperation of finding meaningful income, I still could not take on an industry where I did not feel secure in rendering accurate and meaningful diagnoses and treatments. The science behind alternative medicine was just not there yet, I felt. I left with only a few days of work in two of the only places that hired me. Not having a stable marriage despite trying and not having a decent medical job can send you into a dark place. Depression tends to win the game and make things worse. Almost half of my classmates had already secured jobs by the time they graduated, and I was still trying to find anything nine months after graduation.

The Struggle is Always Real: Unexpected Solutions in Unexpected Sources

It was a dark time in my life. I was in and out of court for various reasons relating to a failing marriage, and I felt like I was hitting a brick wall repeatedly. In these times, I can see why many people seek the comfort of a bottle or a drug, but I grew up with bottles and the drugs around me, and this was not a viable option. One day, while taking a bus to an appointment, I saw a random physician assistant's name on a sign posted outside of an unassuming office building on Hillside Avenue in Queens.

Now imagine 10 lightbulbs going off simultaneously in the mind of a person in desperation. I knew I had to seize the opportunity and call that office that day. It was very shortly after seeing the PA's outdoor office sign that I called and pretended to be a friend of a friend from the physician assistant's alma mater and proceeded to ask him for references or any help finding a PA position. From our interaction came two leads for a potential hire, a hospital, and a single physician-owned orthopedic clinic in Brooklyn, NY. Brooklyn kept pulling me back in!

That was the first day of my professional life created through quiet thinking and initiative. Orthopedics was not my first choice, but my first love. It wasn't an easy road, and I had to make temporary pivots that may not have always aligned with my career goals before landing my second love: Medical Aesthetics.

Looking back, I'm grateful for the challenges I faced because they made me stronger and more resilient to failures, and there were many more to come. I hope my story can inspire others to never give up on their goals, no matter how difficult the path may seem; strength comes from perseverance.

Entrepreneurship and Technique: The Inception

After gaining enough experience with the healthcare system, I created an outsourcing medical-personnel agency catering to the pain specialties (orthopedics, neurology, pain management, and physiatry). This all started about two years after my employment, and I had the pleasure to meet and hire the most wonderful PAs, nurses, and LPNs to fulfill this dream. It went exceptionally well; the business strategy and the need it filled were necessary at the time. I took advantage of the leisure time my new business afforded me.

Golf became a source of time for introspection, especially the driving range where the technique of the swing in the game puts you against yourself. Here was the beginning of understanding how important technique is to accomplishing a consistent routine for predictable results. The act of repeatedly performing the same successful combination of moves repeatedly will allow consistency in the desired response over time until you can predict the outcomes. Hence my career-long professional mantra: "Technique + Consistency leads to Predictability."

This period of success and comfortable living was not meant to last. Adversity is like a cold winter's draft blowing ever so quietly through the windowsills that always finds a way in and so life seems to become a series of never-ending tasks of overcoming hurdles. Well, I lost it all in part due to a lengthy divorce but more precisely from not foreseeing and planning well enough to protect myself and my company from such a catastrophe.

There were also the highly fraudulent activities that the pain specialties seem to attract which did not align with my values or my reason for becoming a medical practitioner. I had to sell everything: a newly constructed home, all physical assets, and later was forced to file for bankruptcy. I started over from zero: zero in my bank accounts, zero friends, zero business, and zero resources to recuperate. Such is life!

I started working again part-time with several different physicians to diversify my skills in the pain specialties. One of these skills was the ability to offer near-pain-free intra-articular injections of the neck, back, shoulders, knees, hands, and feet. This was a major exposure to the art of the injection with precise placement of the needle into the joints to facilitate a pain-free experience for the patient. I began to lose interest in medicine, however, due to the abundance of unnecessary surgeries, X-rays, MRIs, pain medications, and medical devices being prescribed to patients for pure financial gain. Medicine was truly a business, a noble business, however it was easily corrupted with the temporary ailing reprieve for some and cures for very few.

The Allure of the Beauty Industry and the Business of Desire

At the height of my discouragement with the medical business and industry, I stumbled upon a yellow flier just lying quietly in a corner and advertising for a Botox™ training course. So I said, "why not?" and I decided to attend. The Botox™ training course made me realize that cosmetic medicine was an art that required creativity, a lot of technique, and a thorough understanding of facial expression. This felt like another path to something I desired and which I hoped and prayed for upon my graduation six years prior. I had a reason now to transition from pain management specialties to cosmetic medical aesthetics. At this point, only dermatologists and a handful of surgeons were tinkering with the idea of Botulinum toxin treatments as a standard beauty treatment, and there were very few articles available in the U.S. to truly learn the intricacies of cosmetic medical treatments.

After a few more training courses of botulinum cosmetics under my belt, I first began treating friends and their families as well as dabbling in concierge house calls and hosting Botox parties. The income necessary to cover the cost of the cosmetic products and pay the essential bills was not enough, to say the least. I had since revised my orthopedic and pain management working hours to invest more time into providing cosmetic treatments; now, my salary was nearing half of my previous income, but the potential was there, and that was good enough for me.

The Botox concierge services were becoming challenging, and after a few years, I realized I needed to open my own physical brick and mortar practice to make an adequate living from my new venture in cosmetic medicine. This is where another Ah-Ha moment came to me; I needed to go where the women were. At the time, women comprised nearly 100 percent of the Botox™ treatment clientele, so the next step ahead was not my favorite, but I decided to rent a room in an existing facial and hair salon. One location became two, and it was at the second location that my medical beauty business model took off. I was working six days a week leaving Sundays to spend quality time with my son who was now 12 years old and living quite far away. Sacrifices were made to accommodate the realities of life around me and with sacrifice, much is lost but much is also gained. I started to see a light at the end of the tunnel, thereby slowly leaving my torrential past behind and looking forward with even more determination. After all, how many times can you reinvent yourself?

The facial and hair salon, Natura Spa, that I leased my treatment room from was quite modern and designed in great taste, bringing the unique styles and flavor of Brazil to New York. The beauty of the spa and the people took the sting out of venturing from the standard medical industry of pain specialties into a specialized facial treatment paradigm I call medical beauty. While working within Natura Spa and Hair Salon was not optimal for my perceived place in medicine, it was providential, as it allowed me to meet my second wife, an amazing woman who has worked tirelessly and stuck by my side as I began to rebuild my life, my career, and my peace.

Reshaping Dreams: Forging Destiny

Finally, I decided to take the plunge and open my own brick-and-mortar medical aesthetic practice, but this was an expensive and daunting task. I had to learn how to operate and manage the business and employees within this new medical beauty industry. There was no precedent to decide what I should or should not do. There were no independent physician assistant businesses I could ask critical questions, so I was on my own again to navigate the path and grow cautiously; however, finding patients, hiring staff, and dealing with state regulations and permits wasn't what I loved to do.

This is where the help of my wife stepped in. We opened our medical beauty practice, and I was finally able to extensively work on my new innovative techniques. This new challenge taught me the value of persistence, resilience, and determination. Dreams can be reshaped at any time, no one has to have a dream and stick to that one dream all their life, but with every dream, the goals to succeed must align with your values if you are to be comfortable and at peace with your business decisions.

With excitement and eagerness in hand, the next journey was already on the way. I was delighted when I discovered a profound passion for the beauty treatment industry and the ability to define the way the business would be operated. A deep sense of integrity and morality for the people looking for physical and psychological positivity kept knocking. Medical beauty was a field that resonated with me on multiple levels, allowing me to combine my innate sense of beauty with a desire to make a positive impact on people's lives. The idea of helping individuals enhance their natural features and regain their confidence ignited a fire within.

One crucial aspect that distinguishes my approach in the medical beauty field is my natural empathetic nature. Understanding the emotional journey that individuals undertake when seeking aesthetic treatments. I strive to create a safe and supportive environment for my clients by listening attentively to their concerns, fears, and aspirations. I aim to build a trusting relationship that allows for open communication and tailored care. We are dealing with real people and real concerns, though a veil/curtain is always held up for them to shield and protect their fears from our sight. For success in this industry, these qualities must be present. People's psychological being is attached to their perception of the physical being, at least the ones who present themselves to us.

The inherent engineering ability developed during my tumultuous high school years was critical in my understanding of human facial anatomy and it was not a coincidence as I learned a few years ago while returning to Barbados on a short family visit. I was told by my aunt about my family's rich history of being engineers in different fields. Of notable significance was my great grandfather's history well before the 1950s when the name "Vanderpool," which was unique on the island, was the head ship's mechanical engineer. I was told about my uncle - also a Vanderpool - who traveled continuously between the islands of the West Indies as the top mechanical engineer for engines of all types.

In the ever-evolving field of medical beauty, staying at the forefront of innovation is crucial. Dedication to continuous learning and professional development, attending conferences, workshops, and seminars to refine our skills and broaden our knowledge by creating venues for other practitioners to learn and share experiences are necessary. By embracing the latest techniques and technologies, medical beauty practitioners can offer clients cutting-edge treatments that deliver optimal results for lengthy periods of time.

THE LUST FOR MEDICAL BEAUTY

Each day in practice feels like a new chapter, filled with diverse individuals seeking their own unique transformations. It is a privilege to be part of their journey, witnessing their confidence bloom as they rediscover their inner and outer beauty. Whether it's sculpting facial features, rejuvenating skin, or refining body contours, I am fueled by the joy of helping my clients achieve their aesthetic goals and regain their self-assurance.

Transformations: Evolving Beautifully in Ways Our Parents Could Only Imagine

Medical beauty offers every client the chance to experience the profound impact that changing some minor physical negatives they may see in the mirror has on them. Beauty, empathy, and engineering in a medical beauty practitioner can have a transforming effect on the way the patient sees themselves and come to appreciate the fleeting nature of physical beauty they carry in their lives. Physical beauty, for many, is an asset, like gold and diamonds; many lives are changed by the value beauty brings with it. I am committed to honoring this industry, exploring new possibilities, and embracing the future advancements that will shape the field of medical aesthetics especially if clients continue to be pleased with the work they allow us to do.

In this ever-evolving industry, my aesthetic colleagues who share similar values, are determined to be a source of inspiration and empowerment for clients, guiding them towards their unique transformations. This statement is very important since it speaks about the need to step into the patient's shoes for a brief moment to truly understand their requests. This allows us, with every treatment, to strive to create an experience that goes beyond physical enhancement and thus leave a lasting impact on the client's self-esteem, physical appearance, and psychological well-being.

Unleashing the Creative Potential: Reflections on Diversity

How do you create a business title/name that reflects the heart and soul of your company? Diamonds, though not the rarest of gems, are by far the most beautifully accepted element that we attach to beauty, femininity, and perfection. Now, there are four distinct groups of facial features that we all are accustomed to if you are observant enough to witness them daily and which have nothing to do with the amount of aesthetic work necessary for beauty, how beautiful the facial features are, or how much aesthetic work is necessary to maintain the beauty of individuals.

These four major facial groups are your 1- Black facial features that have a high amount of prominent projections, striking lines, and angles to the face 2- Asian facial features that converge into a more smooth and roundness that communicates with each other forming a congruent set of gratifying fullness 3-White facial feature that lend to a more elongation and harmony between angles, lines, and curves, and 4- Latino facial features that tend to blend the above features in a gorgeous homogeneous set creating a completely different look. These four facial features are not separate and due to the migration and travel of human beings for thousands of years, there are hybrids within each particular group. These four facial features respectively correspond to the four diamonds within our logo.

As the lead designer for our Diamond Works Medspa media kit, I was tasked with creating a logo that would capture the essence of our brand. After considerable and careful consideration, it was decided to develop the multifaceted four-diamond-flowered logo that would reflect the unique differences within each client's facial features. After all, the entire business of beauty is about the client.

The four diamonds of the logo, being the accents of our logo, represent the idea that every diamond has its own remarkable features that makes it unique just like us. Every face has its beauty to be interpreted by the viewer and until that rough diamond is cut, shaped, and polished, like our faces, many times, the real beauty that makes the individual beautiful without the work done is missed.

Even if the cuts of the diamonds are made by one expert gem-cutter also known as a lapidarist, each diamond cannot be the same and will never be identical. They cannot reflect light the same way. Similarly, the faces of identical twins are never exactly alike. Our overall shape, our angles, our edges, and finally our facets determine the beauty we all seek to attain, and the way the ambient light bounces off the facial feature makes the difference. Therefore, our logo's diamonds represent the unique beauty that all four major facial feature groups possess.

The petals present as the centerpiece of the logo have two colors - a darker green and a light green, reflecting different tones of the skin's color. Everyone's skin has different tones, though, less likely in albino skin, which is void of melanin. These lighter colors bloom out of the darker background color, the rich maturity of the darker green gives an ambience to the lighter green, representing growth, renewal, and reinvigoration. Medical beauty should also be about helping our clients enhance and revitalize their natural beauty through their skin tone. The petals in our logo are a reminder that we are here to help our clients renew and reinvigorate themselves, just like a flower that blooms anew.

In conclusion, our multifaceted four-diamond-petaled logo captures the essence of our brand. It represents the unique beauty of the four distinct facial features - the diamonds - the growth and renewal being offered, and the organic nature of our clients' faces (the petals). At Diamond Works Medspa, we are committed to helping our clients enhance their natural beauty while embracing their unique characteristics.

CHAPTER THREE

MEDICAL BEAUTY

The History and Emergence of New World Beauty

1800 - Topicals & Elixirs

Pre-1800s, before the introduction of the hypodermic needle, beauty treatments were insanely limited to external applications of pigment-rich makeups and countless elixirs that were stirred up and consumed in the hopes of a younger, more captivating look.

It was in the early 1800s that a young Dr. Justinus Kerner living in Germany was tasked to find the reason for outbreaks of death following exposure to a favorite ghoulish dish of blood sausages. He was able to discover the causative agent narrowed down to this particular meal, thus was the beginning of a long journey from death to desire in this bacteria called Botulinum Toxin.

1844 - Francis Rynd

During the Victorian era, an Irish doctor was credited with the first recorded injection using a hollow needle. This was at the time of the cholera epidemic, which was devastating Europe at the time. A decade later, Alexander Wood attached a fabricated syringe to that hollowed needle, and beauty medicine took an enormous leap forward.

1850s

Just shortly after the invention of the needle and the syringe attached to the needle, paraffin wax was being experimented with for the correction of age-related hollowness. Paraffin, a residual naturally occurring byproduct of refined petroleum/oil that is a solid at room temperature and liquid at temperatures above 110 degrees. By some fortuitous means, the needle syringe and paraffin wax were married, setting the stage for a new beauty-enhancing solution to topple all others.

The first cosmetic procedure using paraffin wax was not for the face at all, but, you guessed it; for the testicles. The procedure was credited to Robert Gersuny, a surgeon living in Austria with a seemingly large number of patients requiring ball-enhancing regimes. You cannot make this up if you tried! Well, the introduction of paraffin/wax injections for cosmetic purposes quickly gained popularity among the financial well-to-dos, the elites and noble people of the day. The space-occupying mass effect of melted paraffin injections could add volume to the cheeks and other parts of the face and body, where deficits occurred.

1853 - Alexander Wood

One of the most important additions to modern medicine was credited to Alexander Wood, the inventor of the syringe that attached the hollowed needle of Dr. Francis Rynd. Alexander Wood was a Scottish physician who became well known for his morphine administration device among many other contributions to medicine. He was looking for a way to get morphine into local regions of the body without passing through the rest of the entire body to avoid some obvious side effects. Let's take a second to understand the impact this made on the history and progression of modern medicine; just about everything being entered into the body besides entering through the mouth or anus will be administered via a hypodermic syringe-needle combo.

Beauty's Renaissance Era: Old World Remedies to New-Age Marvels

Fat grafting is all too old for us today especially with the introduction of medical tourism where people will visit foreign countries to find a more cost-efficient solution to breast and buttock injections. This practice is typically commonplace today, but not a few hundred years ago.

According to *Seminars in Plastic Surgery*, fat transfer from one body part—the forearm—to the face was accomplished by a German doctor, Gustav Neuber, in the late 1800s. This is one of the earliest known successful autologous fat grafting procedures performed, and it paved the way for a new understanding of cosmetic surgical solutions.

Surgical options were being considered and not just for fixing broken body parts but also when the aesthetics of the face and body is broken, surgery can now be an option. However, due to many failures, the cost of the procedure, and a limited understanding of demonstrating lasting results in the process, autologous fat injections were not as common, and this led to further investigation and research for the perfect remedy. Today, autologous fat grafting still occurs with better long-term outcomes, but consistency and predictability remain a challenge. Fat grafting still remains uncertain in the best of surgical hands, and the longevity of the results is less appealing.

Paraffin's Fall from Grace

When the 1920s arrived, paraffin injections had lost its favor, its unpredictable evolution and massive immunologic responses made it a non-impressive and high-liability risk for both patients undergoing the procedure and surgeons administering this paraffin miracle oil. Unfortunately, the availability of surplus cash and the desperation for looking youthful forced many women to continue taking their chances with risky treatments and riskier practitioners who knew that they did not have enough safety data to support the ongoing use of paraffin injections, and their thirst for money is what ultimately lead to treacherous outcomes.

Paraffin injections had disastrous consequences leading to large abnormal growths within the injected areas of the face and body, obliterating the person's features, and causing unknown tumors that required surgical excision leaving most with facial disfigurements. Surgical excision of the paraffin product from the patient's face became a new commonplace procedure but did not deter the thirst for beauty and resurrecting youthfulness.

As a medical professional, I have seen the devastating consequences of paraffin injections, a beauty treatment that was once touted as the answer to restoring youthful looks. Paraffin, a petroleum-based product, was used in the past to replace the loss of volume in the cheeks and other facial features. Unfortunately, the results were often catastrophic.

Initially, paraffin injections were used as a replacement for animal fat injections. As medical practitioners stopped using animal fat, paraffin became the new go-to substance for restoring volume. The treatment seemed promising initially, but many issues soon started to arise. The side effects of paraffin injections were severe, and disastrous consequences followed. Women who underwent the treatment developed large abnormal growths on their faces, which obliterated their natural features. Moreover, they experienced unknown tumors that required surgical excision, leading to disfigurements. The surgical excision of the paraffin product became common practice, but it did not deter the thirst for beauty and resurrected youth. Women continued to take their chances with risky treatments that did not have much safety data to support their ongoing use.

Silicone: The Rise and Fall of a Promising Remedy

As a medical beauty expert, I have seen many patients in desperation and tears seeking cosmetic treatments to enhance their appearance and restore their youth. Over the years, I have witnessed the evolution and decline of different cosmetic procedures, products, and techniques. One such product that gained immense popularity in the 1940s - 1960s and gradually devolved was silicone injections.

Early uses of silicone injections for body enhancements were by prostitutes in East Asia, notably in Japan, after World War II. Prior to the American occupation of Japan, the women of Japan found no need to artificially enhance their physiques as Asian men liked their natural Asian bodies. However, crass Americans were used to larger breasts, which was not in abundance in Japan, and this started the trend for bigger boobs. Goat's milk was the first option but ultimately failed due to obvious reasons such as contamination, infection, short duration, etc. and then silicone was next with directly injecting into the breast tissue for an "Americano Express."

While silicone did offer the success of size, the price to pay was, again, disfigurement from silicone granulomas, and the breast tissue becoming solid or sometimes gangrenous.

I have seen firsthand the negative effects of silicone injections. While it is true that silicone injections can produce a mass effect, restoring volume in specific locations, the product's unpredictable evolution and massive immunologic response made it a non-impressive and high-liability risk factor for medical practitioners. Silicone injections were also difficult to remove once injected, leading to long-term complications and disfigurements.

Silicone First Accounts and Observations

Today, we still see the effects of silicone injections, with many patients coming to us seeking corrective procedures to address the damage caused by previous injections. Some physicians still use silicone injections, touting their longevity and cost-effectiveness.

However, as practitioners, we need to recognize and address the risks associated with these procedures and ensure that patients have the information they need to make informed decisions. The use of silicone injections for cosmetic procedures remains controversial, with some physicians in the U.S. and abroad still using it as a permanent means of rejuvenation. They promote lifelong longevity with no need to continually spend time and money to remove lines and fix hollows. It is important to remember that humans tend to selectively avoid hearing the risk portion of a consultation and at times, the risks are also hurried over in discussions lured by the promise of restorative beauty.

Clients should be informed of the potential risks associated with any cosmetic procedure, including the use of silicone injections if it is still used in the medical offices they attend. Silicosis (the negative overgrowth effects of silicone injections) can be a painful and disfiguring condition that may take years to manifest. We should prioritize the safety and well-being of our clients and promote responsible decision-making when it comes to cosmetic procedures.

As a medical professional, I strongly advise against the use of silicone injections for cosmetic purposes. The risks of complications and disfigurements far outweigh the benefits of such treatments. It is essential to educate patients on the dangers of these risky treatments and to provide safe and effective alternatives that can restore their youthful appearance without compromising their health and well-being. Beauty should not come at the cost of one's health and life.

The Story of Jennifer

As a medical aesthetic provider, I remember my first encounter with "silicosis lips" early on in my career. At the time, there was no name for what I did. The practice of only injecting facial devices (fillers) was not a recognized specialty. I met Jennifer, a trans female who was looking to rejuvenate her face to look more feminine. She had already undergone body treatments such as fat grafting to achieve a more feminine shape, but her face still looked masculine. She came to me in tears but also in anger, frustrated with the high fees and lack of results from other doctors.

Jennifer's lips were siliconized, which meant that they protruded abnormally and looked like elongated bubbles or outpouching of the pink lining of the lips. I knew I needed to get into Jennifer's head and find out what she wanted and did not want to have. Her priority was to get rid of the silicone implants in her lips. I agreed and gradually, using a radiofrequency/high-frequency laser (rF/hF) began the slow process of scraping little by little the tissue-infused silicone stuck to the fatty portions of the lips. This process is not for the faint of the heart, as it involves burning the silicone and flesh away. The silicone implants integrate so aggressively with the tissue that they become indistinguishable from normal tissue, and removing them can be a painful and challenging process.

The body sees the silicon as an invader and attacks it violently, causing growth in the immediate region along with water retention in the vicinity. This leads to the gradual growth of the injected region, resulting in "pillow lips." Jennifer's lips had this characteristic, sending a message to the viewer of insecurity, ill choices, psychosis, and untrustworthiness. No one wants to display this look, especially a trans person who is always visible to everyone. My goal is to help my clients achieve their desired look while avoiding risky procedures that can lead to disfigurement and insecurity. Injecting fillers is an art form, and I strive for perfection in my work, making 99% of my clients happy with the results.

Getting rid of silicone implants is a feat of difficulty like no other aesthetic corrective procedure. Definitely no walk the park for the patient and practitioner. It's a fiery ordeal where the silicone attacks the flesh and battles it out. The silicone has such a strong bond with the tissue that in many instances you can't tell them apart. It's like they joined forces and became one indistinguishable mass. But here's the redeeming part - the body goes on defense mode toward this foreign substance and starts encircling the silicone like holding a criminal in a prison cell, locked away for eternity or when the body's immune system fighting ability decreases. The weird phenomenon known as "lip pillowing," occurs with this tragic battle between silicone injected and the body's immune defense to persistent foreign body exposure. This can be seen today by many celebrities such as Donatella Versace who still maintains a glimpse of that striking beauty once demonstrated, Lisa Rinna who is still beautiful and captivating minus the poorly restored lip architecture, Angelina Jolie with her marvelous looks still at times seems to present a silicone structured lip with slight pillowing to the outer lateral vermillion, and countless more who were unlucky enough to innocently have their lips injected with silicone before the introduction of hyaluronic acid fillers or by over-zealous medical doctors lacking the keen knowledge of the damage they are actually inflicting for life. Yikes! But fear not, all. Once those lip pillows deflate a bit, it's time for the true makeover magic to work its wonders by some of us well-tuned medical beauty expert injectors. Lip fillers can come to the rescue, redefining your lips definition, angles, symmetry and bringing those natural attributes back to life with a bright and full appearance. So, say goodbye to the unwanted silicone invaders and hello to a rejuvenated and fabulous you, if you unfortunately had silicone injected in the past. And yes, in case you were wondering, we repeated this information on the page because we really want you to understand and appreciate both the pain and the remedy in this process.

The presence of silicon within the body triggers a forceful immune response, which perceives it as a threat and launches a vigorous attack. This aggressive reaction leads to localized swelling and retention of fluids, causing the surrounding area to expand. As a result, the injected region experiences a gradual expansion, resulting in the formation of what's commonly referred to as "pillow lips." Jennifer's lips exhibited this distinctive trait, conveying a message of self-doubt, questionable decisions, psychological distress, and an air of untrustworthiness. This aesthetic is particularly undesirable, especially for individuals who are constantly in the public eye, such as transgender individuals.

My primary objective is to assist my clients in achieving their desired aesthetic while steering clear of potentially hazardous procedures that may result in deformities and a lack of confidence. The administration of fillers is an intricate artistic endeavor, and I am dedicated to achieving excellence in my craft, leading to the satisfaction of 99% of my clients with the outcomes. The removal of silicone implants is an arduous process that involves the controlled dissolution of both the silicon material and adjacent tissue. The silicon adheres so seamlessly to the surrounding tissue that it becomes nearly indistinguishable from the body's natural structures. The body's immune response perceives the silicon as an intruder, prompting an aggressive reaction that gradually enlarges the treated area, giving rise to the formation of the unwanted "pillow lips." Following a significant reduction in this effect, the true rejuvenation process commences, utilizing lip and cheek fillers to restore well-defined lip contours and angles, as well as to enhance the cheeks, ensuring a vibrant and naturally elevated appearance.

Next Runner Up: Botox Beginnings

In the early 1940s, botulinum toxin A (Botox™) gained popularity in the world of medical research through experiments on animals and its inhibition of muscular activity. Botox was also studied as a potentially useful biological weapon in chemical warfare during World War II. Botulinum toxin is a catalyst of sorts that, when ingested (poison) or injected (venom/medicine), inhibits the movement of muscles, hence fewer creases and wrinkles. When used appropriately and on a schedule, it can result in a considerable age-relieving benefit for the patient. Botox™ is technically a drug, venom, and poison used to enhance beauty; it all depends on one's perspective.

In the 50s and 60s, the potential benefits of botulinum toxin began to gain ground, as it was becoming less feared for its unique effects and was materializing into a potential treatment for abnormal eye movements. Botox was first approved by the FDA in 1989 (the year I ventured on U.S. soil) for the treatment of strabismus, a condition that causes abnormal eye movements and impaired vision. This approval indicated that botulinum toxin had become a safe viable option and was no longer associated with the risk of death that was often associated with Botulinum toxin poisoning.

At that time, botulinum toxin was not considered a potential beauty treatment for the masses. Most people, besides the rich, were less occupied with beauty and more concerned with surviving, as the country had just emerged from World War II, a crippling depression, plunged into another major war, and thus a significant reduction in expendable household cash. The median household income today compared to the 1960s and 1970s is approximately 50% higher as measured in 2020 dollars.

However, with the lack of men due to the war, women were entering the workplace and doing jobs that were once reserved only for men. This emboldened attitude of the female population not only towards supporting themselves and family but also taking control of their bodies. Women also became bolder in their thoughts about beauty and fashion, and a new era was thrust upon us.

It's worth noting that botulinum toxin is the deadliest toxin known to man, and ingestion of the toxin is fatal. However, several cases still occur every year in the United States from the ingestion of spoiled or contaminated foods. As with any medical treatment, Botox should only be administered by trained professionals and in accordance with FDA regulations.

In 1989, Botox™ was a revolutionary medical treatment for the management of Strabismus (mal-alignment of the eyes) and Blepharospasm (uncontrolled eyelid twitching). Shortly after the treating physicians noticed that the crow's feet (wrinkles and lines running outward from the lateral corner of the eyes) vanished after Botox™ injections were performed for strabismus and blepharospasm.

This discovery became the true value of Botox Cosmetics™, a new treatment to remove wrinkles and look younger. Later, Botox became a trigger word in the general population signifying the essence of unnecessary vanity as thousands flocked to receive their Botox beauty treatments. Before this time of beauty-enhancing medical treatments, medical and non-medical practitioners used pig's fat, paraffin/wax, and silicone injections to replace the loss of volume in the face, but with disastrous consequences. Allergic and anaphylactic reactions ensued, and such treatments were at times life-threatening, which resulted in the discontinuation of such treatments.

The Art of the Gel

As a medical practitioner, I know firsthand the importance of using the right tools to achieve the desired result. While artists have the luxury of experimenting with different paint brushes to create various styles and gestures, in medical aesthetics, we must rely on the properties of different gel consistencies to create the desired look and to achieve a long-lasting effect.

Hyaluronic acid (HA) gels are popular in medical beauty for facial rejuvenation and youthfulness. However, not all HA gels are created equal. Each gel has its unique chemical and physical properties that can affect the final result and lasting effect once injected into the facial tissue. As a result, there is no one-size-fits-all approach to using these gels. One product may work perfectly for one patient but may be disastrous for another.

Two of the most popular brands of HA gels used in the United States are Juvéderm and Restylane. While the volume of HA and the needle sizes used remains constant, the differences between the two brands lie in their physical and chemical properties, making them ideal for different applications. It's essential to understand these differences to choose the right gel for each patient.

I often compare the different gel types to an artist's paint medium. Each gel has a unique consistency and finish, just like various types of paint. For instance, oil paint has a semi-thick, almost toothpaste consistency and takes a long time to dry, resulting in a smooth or rough surface finish depending on the quantity applied in any one area along with the brush's application. In contrast, water paint is very thin, dries quickly, and results in a non-textured flat finish regardless of how much paint is applied. Then there is acrylic paint that can have a finish of both textured and non-textured, dries quicker than oil paint but not as fast as water paint.

Similarly, HA gels with different consistencies can create various shapes and styles on the patient's face, resulting in different looks desired. As a medical beauty injector, it's essential to have extensive knowledge of these gel types to aide in the prediction of the final result accurately. If a practitioner cannot predict the outcome, there's still more for them to learn.

Medical beauty is art; it requires skill, knowledge, and the right tools to achieve the desired result. While we may not have the luxury of changing needles frequently, we can use different gel consistencies to create unique shapes and styles on the face along with different injection techniques. Therefore injectors must understand the physio-chemical properties of each HA gel to ensure the best outcome for their patients.

Any devoted artist will tell you that you can create many styles, shapes, and gestures using different paint brushes or brush strokes, well, the same is true for HA gels in creating different looks. In medical aesthetics, we do not have the luxury of using many different types of gels at once, however, the styles, shapes, and gestures are created by the use of different gel types.

HA gels, besides just increasing volume, can be used to create shapes, styles, and gestures in the face for rejuvenation and youthfulness.

Since no two products sold in the United States can ever be identical, no two HA gels are made alike. Each HA gel used in medical beauty has different rheologic (physical-chemical) properties, making them do different things in the face once injected. This is why we say one product does not fit all. The two major competing HA gel brands listed earlier are Juvéderm, which is made and manufactured in France and Restylane, which is made and manufactured in Switzerland. There are a few other brands such as Revance-RHA, and Merz-Belotero also being sold and used in the United States. For the sake of simplicity, I will stick to the two major selling brands in the United States, Juvéderm HA gels and Restylane HA gels.

The needles accompanying the HA gels are typically the same size and designed for the ease of use and not necessarily for the remnants of facial medical beauty. This allows for less variation or deviation in patient outcomes for the novice injectors. Many times, depending on the location of the injection, the size of the needle needs to be changed to allow for a desired look and final outcome. Therefore, the needle size becomes a constant in the calculation of optimal results; the more constants you have, the more predictable the outcomes can be, which leads to the understanding that removing as many variables in our techniques allows for happier patients.

Think of the HA gel types as the artist's paint medium. For example: oil paint that has a semi-watery consistency, takes a long time to dry and typically finishes somewhat flat or without much height off the canvas, which can leave a smoother surface finish. Here would be an example of Picasso's early works in cubism and broken bodily features, notably his portraits of the face. Very watery water paint dries very fast and finishes without any height off the canvas leaving a flat smooth surface finish. Here would be an example of many Japanese waterworks such as the famous Katsushika known for his work, The Great Wave of Kanagawa.

Acrylic paint that is not watery at all, but stiffer, and dries in a shorter amount of time, not as long as oil paint and certainly not as fast as water paint, can leave a very rough finish with a lot of height and ridges off the canvas, leaving a heavily textured surface finish called impasto works. Here would be an example of many famous artists such as Rembrandt van Rijn, Vincent Van Gogh, and Willem de Kooning. Acrylic can leave heavily textured surfaces, and this is my favorite type of paint medium to work with.

Depending on the rheologic (physical and chemical) composition of the HA gel, we can create many different shapes on the face thus creating many different looks desired. The intricate knowledge of these HA mediums is necessary to predict the outcome of the patient's face. I often tell my students and interns that "if you cannot predict the patient's final result, there is still a lot of learning to do" and if you are ever concerned about your patient's facial outcome or ever say to yourself, "I hope this treatment comes out well" then yes, there is a lot still to be learned.

As you can see from the timeline of medical beauty, there have been many improvements over time in the medical beauty industry. Thankfully, many of the treatments that have been proven to be dangerous have been dropped from the repertoire of any reputable practitioner. As we look into the future, I am anticipating new and exciting discoveries and improvements for safe facial reconstruction, rejuvenation, and beautifying the face in the field of medical aesthetics.

CHAPTER FOUR

VANITY'S PARADOX
Social Pressures to Pursue and Yet Conceal Beauty

When individuals whom most would consider very attractive hear the word "beauty" directed toward themselves or are addressed as beautiful in conversation, they often dismiss such compliments out of concern for appearing vain. Why is it that we conceal our desire for beauty? Is the criticism of vanity originating from those who are less likely to afford or achieve the very youthful beauty they criticize?

Ask yourself, how many people who strive for perfection of their outer beauty criticize another for doing the same? The number is possibly zero. Seeking inner beauty is more accepted and encouraged than seeking outer beauty for many reasons, one being that inner beauty can be construed as a virtue and relates to healthy responsible living. Physical outward beauty in the Renaissance era (Fourteenth to the sixteenth century) was linked to being virtuous and was considered a connection to the spiritual being who then blessed you with that outward beauty.

Therefore, if someone carried themselves physically beautiful (skin, clothes, or hair) they were thought of or perceived as pure in heart.

Conversely, if one did not have the monetary means to dress in beautiful garments of color or possessed the gift of youthful beauty, they were not as engaged by the ruling members of society: this is the spirit of our beloved Cinderella story." It reminds me today of a popular phrase "No one is ugly, just poor." History tends to repeat itself in many ways. We all have something that we would inarguably love to change about our features, now whether we can afford to change it or have the resources to change it is another story.

So, what is beauty? It is not something you can hold onto and certainly not something we all have eternally. Beauty is a perishable gift belonging to no one for too long, but with enough pampering, nurturing, and the right hands, its allure will remain by our side as a resource for whatever benefit we seek.

First, we don't need aesthetic medicine to save us from the dangers of this world or even for basic survival. Some may argue that their physical presentation, their looks, and their first impression have had a profound change and/or importance in their lives at some point and which may have contributed to a good life for them. I would argue that looks are everything. Human beings have based a majority of their decisions on another's looks initially, whether profiling negatively or positively or just forming a basic judgment toward the other person's character.

If I Am Beautiful, Why Do I Need Work Done?

Of the five main senses that we are aware of and typically speak of, sight is the most used tool when judging an individual, hence on first sight and subsequent interactions. We primarily make our sexual decisions (at least initially) on the type of face attached to the body we will sleep with. The face ultimately determines the sex worthiness of our partners.

We use our vision to form an opinion or judgment on the character of the person presenting themselves to us, at least initially. From an anthropological sense, sight is the main sense that has kept us away from danger. Danger from wild animals, our immediate environment, and other human beings around us. No one wants to lose their sight. How does it feel when you see someone legally blind walking with a blind stick or white cane? How do you feel when you see a very young individual in or around their early 20s walking with a blind stick or white cane? This is a gut-wrenching circumstance that we all shudder at when we think of it. It is the one thing that puts extreme fear in all of us—losing our sense of sight.

We ask ourselves the question, is this person visually pleasing to us? When we say sex sells, and sex in many ways sells everything, it involves looking and making a visual assessment of what is in front of us. So, it is by no means inaccurate that we use our sight to judge others and who they are. The most beautiful model or many of them who have graced the covers of beauty magazines or have been a spokesperson for the beauty industry and all products relating to beauty can point to multiple flaws in their face. I have had many magazine print models in my chair at various times, and I was always in disbelief that the individual can find so many issues with the same face that has propelled them to popularity and success.

The Perfectionism Epidemic: The Role of Social Pressure and Pop Culture

Perfectionism is not only the desire to look immaculate or dress perfectly but also the belief that being perfect in our looks can be achieved. We are in an era of awareness where we see that having medical beauty treatments on the face or body has very little to do with beauty alone but with the awareness of medical beauty's possibilities and taking advantage of the technology for pure gain.

I often tell my friends and colleagues that I don't sell Botox or fillers, but everything else surrounding the variables leading to beauty such as confidence, self-esteem, a sense of symmetry, and evenness, which equates to refinement and youthfulness. Beauty is ethereal. It is here today and gently gone tomorrow or at times, gone as quickly as it arrives before it is recaptured again (depending on the lighting environment you are in).

Pop Culture's Influence on Beauty

So, unlike happiness, we can reach beauty, but it'll leave you one day, eventually.

Popular culture dictates the scene of the era. The 70s were all about freedom and psychedelics; in fact, this era was defined by the infusion of LSD into mainstream ideology creating a fantasy world within this world. Flared pants and platform shoes skimmed across the disco lounges— Studio 54 anyone? The only real cosmetic (medical or not) changes one could make were new makeup colors, colorful loose-fitting clothing, and breast implants, which were all the rage.

The 80s came in with the working girl and shoulder pads, and movies and television featuring more women and more lead women in roles like Charlie's Angels. Video games portrayed strong muscular female characters kicking male butts like Street Fighter. This time it was laced with women taking charge of their bodies and displaying them in whatever manner they chose: Triple D and F breast engorgement was a thing and fat grafting was also becoming popular.

The 90s gave us the rise of the internet, which permeated throughout the entire world one country at a time bringing everyone together, but not. The 90s was considered a relatively peaceful time without the stain of the cold war on our backs. Nirvana, Evogue, Destiny's Child, and Spice Girls all gave us "Girl Power" furthering the sense of strength and power in many of our leading women of today.

When describing the art of medical aesthetics, I prefer to use statements about facilitating the means to the journey of one's beauty. An analogous way to look at beauty is that your face is like a slow-moving 3-D canvas and everything the injector artist does to your face is fleeting, therefore, careful work must be done to support the features that are still present in the face as well as creating new features that complement the existing face.

Every tissue and structure in the face constantly moves, and constantly changes and some regions move faster than others at different rates and directions of movement depending on the tissue type. Another way to look at the job of a medical aesthetic injector is to imagine a bust of a person's head and face made out of soft clay that is pulled by gravity. The forehead and brow slowly drift downward, the nose either falls fatter or begins to cave in at the tip, the cheeks always fall flat and wide, the jawline disappears under the weight of the middle and lower cheeks, and the lips twist and bend out of its perfect orbital shape.

My job is to anticipate the facial features that will fall first due to dermal hints as well as correct the already aging facial features. Your face continuously changes over the course of weeks to years and sometimes even days. Yes, many features and structures "go south" so to speak, and we typically say gravity is taking over, however, the bones don't go south, the ligaments don't go south, the hairline doesn't go south, so different structures do different things as time passes based on my 4 S's of visual skin aging.

My 4 S's of Visual Skin Aging

1- SUN - the sun is undoubtedly the most direct cause of visual damage to the surface of the skin. Although there are three type of ultraviolet radiation produced: ultraviolet - UV-A, UV-B, and UV-C, it's the UV-A that causes the most damage being emitted more continuously throughout the day than the other UV radiations. UV radiation directly causes destruction to the DNA of the skin cells, which forces the cells to repair constantly leading to potential errors in DNA transcription and likely cancer or cell death. As the skin cells die, the overall thickness of the skin layers thins, allowing creasing from underlying muscle movement.

2- STRESS - Cortisol levels rise when the human body is under mental or physical fatigue. The adrenal glands will release enough cortisol to increase your body's sugar level for potential boosting of the energy level regularly. This process helps the body perform better in tight situations like when you are studying at the last minute for that important test, or when you must run or fight for your life. Increased cortisol will also increase sebum production leading to blackheads and clogged pores, a disruption in the skin barrier, and a change in the normal bacterial flora of the body all leading to poor skin health and ultimately, an aged looking skin.

3- SLEEP - Sleeping on the face or the side of the face will undoubtedly create early creases in the skin due to the 12-14 lbs. of pressure over several hours upon the facial skin. The weight of the head is similar to the weight of an average watermelon, just under 15 lbs. Imagine this weight crushing your cheeks toward your nose and mouth causing vertical or diagonal lines running up and down the face. These are called sleep lines, and they do indeed become permanent over time.

Besides the lines, you are stretching the skin considerably every day 6-9 hours per day, 365 days per year. That translates to 2,190 to 3,285 hours of skin pulling and stretching. Now, say I came to your workplace for one hour each day and rested my palm on the side of your face and gently pulled downward continuously for that one hour. You will never go for it; however you do this over 2,000 hours every year. Physical skin stretching will result in early upper eyelid hooding, early jowls, and turkey necks. No one wants that.

4- SOAP - Washing the face every day is by far an easily prevented skin aging habit. Soaps break down the natural oily protective layer of the facial skin thus rendering the skin vulnerable to any level of UV radiation from the sun or fluorescent light bulbs. This drying out of the skin with soap also leads to chronic dry skin problems such as acne, rosacea, telangiectasias (tiny red spider vessels on the face), and micro cracks interrupting your normal protective skin barrier. The first thing we all were taught to do every morning is to get up and wash our face. Now, I do not know about you, but my pillow case is always clean before I lay down to sleep and at no point in time does my face get dirty requiring a soapy sudsy wash. When you awaken your face is still clean and does not need over washing. Just rinse the face with warm water first, then cold water and your skin will thank you by looking its best and its youngest.

Fat-Filled Faces and Aging Gracefully

The skin tends to slouch, stretch and elongate as it becomes thinner and lighter at which point gravity has taken over pulling these structures down. Facial fatty tissue, depending on its location in the face, can either become smaller with age or soft and looser thus not being able to support its weight any longer. Case in point, beautiful people with full luscious cheeks regret their natural fullness as soon as the medial and middle fat pads in the cheeks starts its gradual descent creating nasolabial folds and creases, marionette lines, and jowls.

By the 30s and 40s, the highest point/curvature of those cheeks has noticeably deflated despite your best intentions of maintaining them. To explain it simply, the superficial fatty cheeks are attached to the underside of the facial skin and are rolling from the inside downward pulling the natural outside curvature of the outer skin inward; this is how lines and wrinkles of the cheeks are initially created.

Let's look at the consistency of fatty tissue within the face. Imagine you are at a kitchen counter with two whole chickens ready to be prepared. First, you cleave into fresh chicken #1, removing some of the fatty areas within that chicken. You notice that the fat of chicken #1's fatty tissue feels and looks dense, full, orange, tough, and can hold itself up on the counter. Next is chicken #2, you cleave into it and notice that the fatty tissue is softer, less orange, looser, and cannot support its weight by flattening out on the countertop.

Chicken #1 is the younger chicken since younger fatty tissue is wholesome and tough and able to stand on the countertop supporting its weight. This is the same fatty tissue within our faces. When we are younger, our faces are full of dense, tough, and rich-looking fatty tissue. As we age, the fatty tissue changes to a less dense, less tough fatty tissue.

The youthful fatty tissue underneath the skin applies pressure against the dermal layer, effectively eliminating any wrinkles or lines on the face. Imagine a fully inflated beach ball without any creases on its surface. Now, gradually deflate the beach ball, and you will observe some areas loosening first, followed by the formation of a few creases.

This phenomenon is why younger faces have fewer wrinkles; however, as we become older, we see a gradual deflation in our fatty tissue with loss of size and volume. The analogy of the beachball holds as you take the air out of the beach ball, the surface of the beachball begins to sag, wrinkle, and lines are formed. The density of the facial fatty tissue no longer holds up or pushes up against the undersurface of your skin with as much pressure as when you were younger.

Also, as the skin becomes thinner with age, lines are easily formed reflecting what's happening below the surface of the skin and within the skin itself. So, the next time you cut into a piece of chicken, observe the fatty texture and try to determine if that chicken was younger or older.

Our Unique Beauty, Signature, and Style

One's beauty should not be seen by a medical aesthetic practitioner as a rigid set of lines, angles, and curves but as a designable malleable mold of delicate clay entrusted in our hands. As we become older, we retain and maintain our beauty that we find acceptable from the perception of ourselves.

However, a different type of beauty gradually and steadily emerges over time. A more mature distinguished beauty: a primary example is George Clooney who had been a very handsome younger man and is now a more distinguished-looking handsome older man. Also, there is Cate Blanchett with such a remarkably beautifully defined face and features and as she's becoming older, the mold of her face continues to bloom. Kate has a very charismatic mature signature look about her that distinguishes her from a typical pretty woman, but this is leading to a very subjective path.

A younger person cannot have matured beauty because the structures that lend to a mature face are hidden behind loads of fatty tissue and muscle within the younger face This is why we can gauge age relatively within one to two decades of a person's chronological age without being too specific. You will never see a 22-year-old's face looking matured and distinguished and you will never see a 52-year-old face looking 20ish full of volume and cuteness.

We all have a discernible signature way of aging that's characteristic of our own and have an algorithmic schematic from an engineer's standpoint. As a beauty expert who has seen thousands of faces a year, I can tap into some of the secrets of the visual aging face and find little pearls of clues and cues that are significant to making someone look younger without gross manipulation of their facial features by the use of overexpanding fillers, dermal threads, and freezing their muscles with Botox.

Recapturing someone's beauty with small amounts of medical aesthetic products in a combination of small precise touches and locations makes subtle changes immensely attractive. Gently subtle but impactful modifications with the use of Botox, fillers, or dermal soft threads are all one needs to recapture their allure or the reason why they loved themselves.

If you don't consider yourself beautiful, then work needs to be done on a physical, psychological, and spiritual level. We are all beautiful and have the same issues, just at different times in our life and different places on our bodies, That statement does not mean that to be beautiful you need medical intervention, but that if there's anything about your physical appearance that leads to a negative feeling within you, there's always something that you can do about it but first you must ask yourself whether that problem is occurring because of how you feel or how others feel about you.

If it is indeed an issue that could be rectified easily, for example forehead lines or lip lines, then by all means if it improves your appearance and it improves the positivity that others see in your features, then it should be done. We fix/alter/modify and change our hair, nails, makeup, and other external features others see and as technology is changing rapidly, this is just another feature of our bodies over which we can gain some control.

If you feel you are beautiful then that beauty, like your house, lawn, or hair needs to be maintained because beauty will never stay with you. Your sense of beauty may stay with you for a long time but your actual physical outward beauty, without the psychological attachment, means that what others see and the positiveness they see by looking at you falters with time. The negative they may see by low or ill maintenance while looking at you can create an unfavorable impression in the viewer's eyes. Your beauty is not only attached to how you feel but how other people feel about you.

For example, if you believe you are the most beautiful person in your immediate surroundings but as you walk among your friends and acquaintances, people look at you less than positively, that at some point will trigger some thoughts in your mind to address what you consider as beautiful and this has nothing to do with your confidence, this has everything to do with reality along with how you feel about yourself.

Deceptive Reflections: Who Do You Truly See

We human beings cannot see ourselves as others see us. We will always be subject to the impression of others with our image. A mirror gives you a kind of two-dimensional view of yourself, but the brain makes out the curvatures associated with that 2D image from the mirror you are looking into. Your brain connects the dots to create curvatures and symmetry. When someone looks at you, they are seeing a 3-dimensional moving image of your face, not a 2-dimensional image. The brain of the onlooker does not have to connect dots to create curvatures about you so they see you slightly differently than when you see your 2-dimensional self in a reflective surface.

This is the very reason we do not like to see ourselves on video, it is then a moving 3-D image that we have never seen and so at the first sight of ourselves on video, we tend to react in the negative, especially if the lighting is not flattering. We never have the real picture of our face in our minds but an image representing our face after our brain has done the work to connect the curvatures, lines, and angles turning the 2-D into a 3-D image.

This is why many beautiful people don't see themselves as beautiful, and we are dumbfounded by how the most beautiful individuals cannot see their own beauty. Our beauty is also structured and taught to us by our environment, our history, and what society deems as beautiful from a young age. This is why sometimes it's hard for us to change our hairstyle or our face makeup or a particular way in how we dress even though the trends continue to change. This is also why so many people love a nostalgic appearance or harken back to a younger time and reminisce by buying retro clothing because that was the time they saw themselves as the most beautiful, especially within themselves. The perception of beauty can be all-encompassing and misleading so we rely on others for their judgment.

If you consider yourself beautiful then there's a certain level of apprehension, you will have as you're becoming older and some of you more than others. I have found that the most beautiful girls tend to have a harder time observing their aging because of the amount of loss they are predicting or witnessing themselves. This is slightly different if the individual who is getting older, loses their beautiful features but is in a committed relationship. A committed relationship will change the way we perceive ourselves and how often we reevaluate the loss.

Sometimes we witness individuals who were once incredibly attractive entering into a committed relationship, only to see their beauty diminish over time. Beauty itself is neither inherently good nor bad; it simply exists. As humans, we tend to categorize things as good or bad to better comprehend and represent our reality, albeit with limited success.

The truth is that reality and everything in the universe transcend the notions of good or bad. We are all interconnected with the universe, and therefore, through deductive reasoning, we too are beyond such judgments. However, assigning good or bad to aspects of life aids society and communities in living together peacefully and cohesively. It's merely a means of organization. Is someone being beautiful inherently good or bad? Is someone lacking beauty good or bad? The concept of good or bad has not been inherently linked to beauty yet. Nevertheless, it is an undeniable truth that beauty often receives rewards, both from others and, more significantly, from ourselves.

A Slow Vanishing Act: The Invisibility of Aging

As we become older, we experience invisibility. Case in point, when was the last time you spoke to someone older than 60 that was not a friend or family member or that you didn't previously know? Many of us tend to see past an elder or through them, although, we may acknowledge the old person, we may greet them, but we do not indulge in conversation, and we do not stick around.

I believe this is an unconscious action we perform and therefore we seldom know we're doing it. To be old is to be alone in your thoughts;

however, to a younger person, the word alone means something different to the older person. The elder have done most of what the younger person has done and so without the physical strength to continue doing more and different things, the mind takes over and the mind cannot contend in its adventures if bothered too much. Grandpa may be grumpy because he is content with his thoughts.

Think of others 10-20 years younger than yourself, do you still want to be doing as much as they are doing? The answer is likely no, you will be content doing things amenable to your age and affordable to your physical endurance. Older people may express the difficulty of being alone, but they will never want much comradery as someone two decades younger.

Older people become invisible, especially individuals younger than 20 years of the elders' age. I once had a patient in my treatment chair with whom I had the same or this very conversation and as I began my discussion on being older and more accurately looking older, which leads to invisibility, she started to cry. I felt so bad about imposing these thoughts upon her. She knew what I was saying was accurate, and she nodded her head in affirmation. I still pressed on with the discussion because she started to discuss many issues with being old. She was not depressed, as she lived with her family, but the sense of being the only one old enough and wise enough alienated her. We both enjoyed this very important discussion; if you're not ready to look old, there is always something that can be done to refresh and rejuvenate, costly or not.

We have the power, the technology, and the devices to do something about visual aging and to look the way we desire. We are designing our faces, and if we choose to not work on our face or our physical appearance, then we will become invisible and maybe sooner than we think. These statements may seem harsh at times, but the reality is most people will rather not tell you are looking old due to the negativity of the statement.

People come to me for beauty advice and treatment and therefore, I am in a peculiar space to discuss with them as gently and empathetic as I can be on the possibilities. This seems like such a taboo topic many days; however, I have not met anyone who did not appreciate my candor. Life is about choices, and the choices you make big or small, subtle or extreme will influence your final destination and what you hope to achieve.

I discuss beautification through medical technologies. I am not speaking of the individuals that overdo their beauty treatments or the practitioners that take advantage of these patients in their vulnerable states, I am speaking about having a reasonable outlook on yourself and expectations of medical technology in reference to your beauty. We change everything about ourselves every day with the use of makeup or hair care products or our clothing and accessories, but when it comes to the face and medical technology, it becomes a little harder to swallow for many primarily because it is new.

Beauty's Dilemma: If I'm Beautiful, Why Do I Need Work Done?

If you consider yourself beautiful, and you should, then like everything else on this planet, maintenance is necessary to delay or evade our harshest critic—time. The most beautiful of us tend to need more work because of the higher expectations from others around them. If you can appreciate how beautiful you are then you can also appreciate the necessity of work to maintain that beauty. Everything shiny, brilliant, dazzling, and ultimately cherished, needs polishing, cleaning, and preserving.

If you love the feel of nice clothing and love to dress to impress, then you understand the cost associated with having the clothing to go along with your personal style. If you are and feel beautiful then you know that it requires more to maintain that feeling about yourself and whether this is a good or bad thing, it does not matter. Therefore, you will need additional work if you wish to cultivate and manage the assets of beauty. This does not mean if you do not manage your beauty, then you are or will not be beautiful because you will age as gracefully as your DNA and self-care determines. My goal is to slow that process down. Everyone appreciates "turning heads," it's a nice confirmation of our looks. However, putting in the extra effort is required.

Conversely, not adding a medical beauty regimen to your upkeep does not strip away your natural beauty. At the end of the day, each person is unique, each person has a specific set of DNA that will stipulate how they age, and each person will have a different perspective on their own beauty (or lack thereof!). So, it is up to each individual to look deep inside themselves and decide what journey is best for them when it comes to medical beauty.

THE LUST FOR MEDICAL BEAUTY

CHAPTER FIVE

HISTORY OF AESTHETICS

Is it Vanity or Simply a Social Need to Belong?

As I immersed myself in the captivating world of enhancing lives via medical aesthetics, I found myself contemplating the motivations behind people of all backgrounds, religions, cultures, and financial status seeking beauty treatments. Is it driven by vanity, a mere pursuit of physical perfection, or is there a deeper psychological need to belong and feel accepted? To understand this complex dynamic, we must explore the historical context leading to medical aesthetics and the cultural influences that shape our perception of beauty.

Throughout history, in the medieval period from the 5th to the 15th century, we have evidence and examples of such art forms including paintings and literature, where humans have sought ways to enhance their appearance. Ancient civilizations like North Africa's Egypt lending their knowledge and customs to Mediterranean countries such as Greece, Italy, France, and Spain to name a few, used cosmetics, ointments, and natural remedies to enhance the features for status while preserving their youthfulness and beauty. These early practices were not solely driven by vanity, but rather by a desire to present oneself in the best possible image and adhere to societal standards of beauty and prestige. However, these early practices were limited by the technology at the time and the lack of safe and effective products/ drugs/potions.

Fast forward to the 14th through 17th century and we have the Renaissance period, where we witness a resurgence of interest in beauty, notably in literature and the arts. Artists like Leonardo da Vinci and Michelangelo celebrated the human form, emphasizing symmetry, proportion, and slowly, the pursuit of idealized beauty. This artistic appreciation of aesthetics and beauty permeated early renaissance society and influenced the way people viewed themselves and others around them. An awareness of individual beauty designs took hold, and this creation of beauty was not only relegated to royalty and the aristocrats, but the everyday peasant woman was also being portrayed in paintings to represent the beauty of the commoner by the great artists.

Beauty Through the Ages: A Historical Context Exploring Medical Standards

We are living in exciting times as the field of medical beauty is evolving, and this compels me to discuss the history of the Barber-Surgeon that changed the history of medicine. We've all heard stories of the original healthcare providers and grave-robbing enthusiasts/anatomists who were foremost barbers and originally ordained by a decree of King Henry VIII to unite the Company of the Barbers and the Fellowship of Surgeons later to be known as the Company of the Barber-Surgeons. The need for medical care of the sick and injured increased exponentially due to the black plague and famine of the 15th and 16th centuries. Treating cuts, wounds, infected limbs, dental extractions, lesion removals, and even amputations was the work of the local barber apprentice-trained layperson.

This profession proved invaluable during times of war, particularly when soldiers found themselves in dire need of medical and surgical care. The individuals practicing barbering in the 14th and 15th century could never have anticipated the profound impact they would have on the advancement of medical practices we witness today. Contemplating the future of medical beauty, one wonders how this field will evolve in the next hundred years. Who will be entrusted with performing medical esthetic treatments? What will be the prevailing credentialing standards and protocols governing this domain? It piques our curiosity to envision the technological advancements and astonishing breakthroughs that may transpire within the next century.

Customarily, we tend to assume that the present situation will remain unaltered and our establishments impervious to change. However, monumental transformations often emerge from seemingly insignificant catalysts. Presently, we find ourselves situated at the vanguard of medical beauty, and it is crucial to acknowledge that everything we experience and observe today will contribute to the emergence of an entirely distinct sector in the future like changing our faces entirely and unrecognizably as easy as changing our shoes.

In the 20th century, advancements in science and technology revolutionized the field of medical aesthetics. The discovery of Botox, dermal fillers, and other minimally invasive procedures offered new possibilities for individuals to enhance their appearance without resorting to surgical interventions. As these treatments became more accessible, they garnered both excitement and controversy but ultimately change is inevitable.

Critics argue that the rise of medical beauty reflects a society obsessed with superficiality and unrealistic beauty standards. They view the pursuit of allurement as a symptom of vanity and self-indulgence, driven by the pressures of media and societal expectations. While it is true that some individuals may seek aesthetic treatments purely for superficial reasons, it is important to recognize that there is often a deeper psychological motivation at play both positive and negative. A psychological motivation that we all share, but lose gradually for a host of personal, interpersonal, age-related, societal, and reasons.

Humans are social creatures, deeply influenced by our interpersonal relationships and the desire to belong. Even those that venture to live outside of the grid still want to be accepted. We strive to fit into societal norms and to be accepted and validated by all others. In a world where appearance is often equated with success, the pressure to conform can be overwhelming. Medical beauty treatments, for many, become a means to boost self-confidence and align with perceived present-day ideals of beauty.

Traditional Medicine vs Medical Aesthetics: Exploring Ingenuity vs Convention

In Western medicine, there are ways that we treat the body to avoid burdensome regiments and delay treatment outcomes. We want expeditious gold-standard treatment regiments to remove the things that can cause problems like misdiagnosing by guesswork, delay healing and recovery by unnecessary treatment, and poor or inadequate treatment products like medical devices and prescription medications.

In standard Western medicine, a series of medical treatment protocols are utilized for efficiency. A protocol is a system of rules/steps governing a particular response to a medical inquiry or a presenting medical problem from a patient. This is what medicine is today and what is taught in medical school; students can memorize and regurgitate the information they are taught. The obvious benefit to protocols is the removal of erroneous treatment regiments ordered by inadequate practitioners and the efficiency of reproducibility; it takes out the guesswork but unfortunately also hinders critical thinking, innovation, and progression.

Medical practitioners are taught in school to follow many sets of protocols necessary for expeditious discharge whenever a patient enters the hospital. There is a certain comforting beauty to these protocols although they can lead to prompt diagnosis, speedier recovery, and established treatment outcomes for patients. This is great when you're forced to see 40 to 60 patients per day, less thinking is involved, and more protocols help speed things along. The downside is that if a protocol is inadequate or wrong, then every patient entering that hospital's protocol will receive the wrong treatment plan leading to vast amounts of patient morbidity and mortality.

Medical protocols can be useful, but they can also become problematic when healthcare practitioners solely rely on them. Protocols often lead to a standardized, one-size-fits-all treatment for all patients, resulting in a kind of mass-produced medicine. The other drawback of excessive reliance on protocols is that it overlooks the need for individualized care, as these protocols may not always be updated, causing harm to the majority over extended periods. Initially, everything may seem satisfactory, but eventually, issues arise especially if capitalistic ideals surpass the virtues of care.

Many healthcare professionals hesitate to challenge the status quo when change becomes necessary, fearing the repercussions or finding the process of implementing change to be burdensome, unfulfilling, or disruptive to their comfortable work environment. After all, change demands effort and commitment.

Aesthetic medicine is somewhat unlike standard medicine, which comprises cardiology, neurology, orthopedics, primary care, OB-GYN, etc. These are the major medical specialties in standard medical practice but aesthetic medicine, which is the cousin of standard medicine, cannot function artistically well with protocols and can be deemed adequate. In medical aesthetic treatments, we most certainly are not treating standard diseases of the body or standard issues that eventually everyone presents with. Standard diseases can be thought of as one dimensional or linear path of treatment where if a person presents to the doctor with this issue, then do this (obviously simplified) and in due time, all protocol treatments become linear except for when the doctor has to start thinking outside of the box or protocol.

Medical beauty is more about the art of the patient's satisfaction as opposed to temporarily alleviating a specific disease like high blood pressure or diabetes or reducing the expression or suffering of a specific ailment or illness. Medical beauty is more of a three-dimensional paradigm where the problem at hand is of an individual issue that some or many people will have, but a situation that everyone will present with: visual signs of aging.

The treatment here is certainly not linear since your ultimate goal is not what the practitioner believes to be beautiful, but what the patient believes or desires for their beauty whether that is in line with the practitioner's view or not. The ultimate treatment or satisfaction of treatment does not really end or reach an end point but rather dwindles slowly as time/aging never stops.

In the realm of Medical Beauty, I find myself immersed in a creative sector that deviates from the conventions of standard medicine. Here, our focus is not on fixing perceived problems, as aging itself is not a problem or a cause for shame. Instead, it is an acknowledgment and appreciation of the cumulative experiences that shape one's life and face—an attitude of discerning what one desires versus what one wishes to avoid. Consequently, our approach differs from that of standardized medicine, as we are not primarily concerned with identifying and diagnosing specific issues. Rather, we aim to offer enhancements that amplify and celebrate the unique expression of everyone's beauty.

We can't simply go into the face and fix fat loss, fat dropping, bone resorption, or ligament laxity. We cannot go into the face and rebuild bone the way it was 20 years ago for that patient, and we certainly cannot go into the face and create the type of thick young fatty tissue and skin that was there 20 years ago. However, we can add enhancements, and in adding enhancements, we can also slow down the visual signs of aging of the individual. This is where surgical face lifts fail, and where Medical Beauty prevails. Medical Beauty is quick, fairly easy for many, and eliminates the extended downtime of surgical procedures. Though there are many instances where surgical procedures are necessary and optimal. Examples are upper and lower eyelid blepharoplasty, excess extended loose skin tissue beyond dermal thread repair, boney reshaping for reduction procedures, etc.

Today's Medical Beauty is not standardized medicine; however, it is treated that way because it was birthed out of standardized medical approaches in treating medical issues such as Botox for strabismus and collagen injections for volume replacement. One day we will separate Medical Beauty treatments from standardized medical treatment protocols as we are thrust into the demand and popularity of this ever-growing creative field of art via innovative biochemical and biophysical devices, equipment, and biomaterials.

The Ambiguity of Vanity: Virtue or Vice

A person's appearance (and their opinion of themselves) is an important concept in the design of life. When you look in the mirror, your perception of your image is what forms a large part of your self-worth, and this underpins a major measure of your personality. So, if you look in the mirror and you wince at what you see, that is motivation, not discouragement, to do whatever is necessary so the image staring back at you is appreciated.

And, of course, the other half of the equation in this design is what other people think of your appearance or presentation. Everyone is judged by another based on the assessment of how visually appealing someone is, what clothes they wear, and what their face looks like. Interestingly, the decision to copulate with another is based initially/primarily, and in many circumstances, only on the facial appeal of the potential bedmate.

The definition of vanity is "an excessive pride or admiration of one's appearance or achievements." Now, we must ask ourselves what the word excessive means. Vanity is a label placed upon others who exercise a higher-than-expected pride or admiration in themselves. Therefore, we are all vain as this quality is part of our 'humanness' but we judge others by the level of care and attention they place in themselves and how much they portray/emit it.

This is expressly similar to being religious but judging others for how religious they portray themselves to be as in "how Jewish are you?" or "You are not Christian enough" or "You are Muslim, how often do you pray?" whether or not they go to Sunday school, whether or not they place their tithings in the usher's tray or how often they read or study the religious scriptures. Our judgments become vices and tools to subjugate, ridicule or put in place others we may not appreciate. As adults, we all have a certain level of vanity, it's a matter of how much vanity is accepted in our immediate circles of influence. As the Proverb says, "Birds of a feather flock together" if you are not accepted among your circle of acquaintances, then you are not of those feathers and should find others who share similar qualities as yourself and who appreciate your choice of presentation.

Vanity is also used as a status symbol. And nowhere is this more apparent than in social media. One of the successes of social media is the ability to look great via filters without having to edit pics, genius! Young people especially are judged by how they appear on their social apps. We live in a society of judging each other's every move. We cannot change that since this has always been a part of any gathering of human beings. The ability to judge others has led to the continuation of our race. Without the ability of our ancestors to make adequate judgments about others, human beings would not exist today. The extension of this phenomenon has led to that judgment being used not for physical survival but also for psychological survival.

Judging or guessing as to a person's character is based upon our history of similarities to that character, whether that history is through social media, television, verbal stories, or our existence and experience with others. We judge to stay alive, however, we also judge our standing in society, where we want to be, where we would like others to be, and what we expect of others. In a society of civilized communities, judging is imperative for our psychological and physical well-being.

Vanity is a complex topic that can be viewed from both positive and negative perspectives. It can be seen as a virtue in the sense that it is a tool used to present oneself in the best possible light and can lead to opportunities for success. On the other hand, it can be viewed as a vice, especially when wielded to manipulate or control others.

The intent behind vanity is crucial in determining whether it is a virtue or a vice. If the intention behind presenting oneself in the best possible light is to create jealousy or to manipulate, it is undoubtedly a vice. However, if the intention is to inspire or make a positive impression, it can be seen as a virtue.

Furthermore, the value of vanity is subjective and dependent on individual circumstances. For those who have the resources to present themselves in the best possible light, there is nothing inherently wrong with doing so. Similarly, for those who cannot afford to do so, it is understandable that they may view such behavior by another with the means to indulge as vanity.

The fear of negative consequences due to vanity is also a real concern. However, it is important to strike a balance between individualism and conformity. While it is essential to embrace one's uniqueness and attractiveness, it is also necessary to avoid excessive exposure that could lead to negative consequences. Your statement is your right as a human being, however, weigh that sentiment with the potential for negative blowback that is unwarranted but is a realistic sequence. For example, wearing expensive jewelry in abundance is your right, but would you do so in a dangerous or unfamiliar neighborhood?

The topic of vanity is complex and multifaceted. It can be viewed as both a virtue and a vice depending on the circumstances and intent behind it. Understanding the value of vanity and striking a balance between individualism and conformity is crucial in determining whether it is a positive or negative trait.

Since we are judged by our appearance and what we present to the world from our physical self we must understand that success begets success or even the perception of success begets success, likewise, beauty begets beauty or the perception of beauty begets beautiful things. Whether we like this or not, it is the way of American life in general and more so, world life in varying degrees.

Vanity is also a tool we can use to ease the burdens of a harsh judgmental society by first ignoring the judges and have-nots since their wishes are irrelevant to your well-being and there's nothing from the have-nots that you are looking to for gain. Vanity has propelled me to the height of my achievements and the way I feel about myself. Most individuals who truly are comfortable and confident in themselves and with what light they present to the world are beautiful though many others would consider them vain.

Striking a Healthy Balance

Spending too much money on facial aesthetic treatments beyond what works is an ongoing problem and tends to be the fault of both the medical provider and the patient. On the provider's end, an over-zealous or greedy aesthetic provider will always push a patient to do most or all of the work necessary for rejuvenation in one sitting. Having all areas of the face done in one sitting allows for a higher charge without the concern of the patient returning, especially if the provider is not sure if the patient will return for additional services based on the results. If a provider-injector does a good job, they will never yearn for patients or use these deceptive practices to draw all the patient's funding in one sitting.

It is unlikely for a patient to spend over $5,000 in one sitting and return to pay more for additional services, so overzealous practitioners will give a one-time quote knowing that the patient will not likely return, and they want to ensure getting as high a bill as possible. At least everything the patient has was spent, and the practitioner can go onto the next unlucky patient. If the medical beauty results are good, the average patient will return for additional services in less than one year; this is not great for some business models in the business of medical beauty where a large one-time fee in one sitting maximizes profits.

These overzealous practices tend to prey on the negative vanity of the patient. Today, the general public knows a lot more about medical beauty than when it first began to emerge in the 50s and 60s. At this point, patients should also be well aware of the practices employed by some medical practices that can trap a patient by playing into the patient's vulnerabilities and level of vanity. Purchasing medical beauty treatments is the same as buying home repair services for your house. There are contractors and there are contractors, just as there are medical beauty practitioners and there are medical beauty practitioners, and wherever there is money to be made, someone will always find a way to take advantage of someone else.

Case in Point

Now, I will preempt this example by saying that not all medical practitioners will stoop to the level of taking advantage of you by participating in the activity of praying on weaknesses. The term "reconstitute" means to reform to a previous state as in rehydrating dried fruits/ food. To re-establish a prior form, for example, to reconstitute botulinum toxin (Botox) to liquid form. The dilute means to diminish the potency/quantity or effectiveness of a liquid product. As professionals, using appropriate terminology is crucial. It is possible to reconstitute Botox and not dilute Botox. We reconstitute Botox (return it to a liquid state) to treat overactive muscles and to reduce or remove lines and wrinkles of the face caused by muscle activity.

Since Botox comes to our medical offices in a white powder form, we must then add normal saline or bacteriostatic water (reconstitute or make it liquid to be transported into a syringe for injection). It is at this stage of preparation of Botox that it can be over reconstituted, which then leads to dilution of the reconstituted product, which will then make its effects diluted = less effective in results and less effective in duration or how long its results will last. Once the Botox is reconstituted, we then quantify the vial into units of measure for reliable measuring of administration.

Here is where it gets tricky, as the Botox "unit" is not standardized! This means that 10 units in one medical spa is not the same as 10 units in another medical spa. You see, the units depend on how the medical spa reconstituted the Botox and if the Botox was diluted (not reconstituted) by adding too much normal saline or bacteriostatic water. Here come the marketing gimmicks: advertising Botox units becomes a form of misinformation to the patient/consumer. How can one medical spa sell Botox for 10 dollars per unit as compared to another medical spa's 15 dollars per unit when the units are not the same? How can the consumer/patient be sure they are getting what they paid for if Botox can be diluted to fit the medical spa's profitability?

This issue becomes apparent when comparing two spas. Let's consider Spa A, which offers Botox at $10 per unit, and Spa B, which is priced at $5 per unit. Although it may seem like Spa B is providing a better deal, it's important to note that their Botox is significantly weaker or diluted compared to Spa A. Spa B's Botox is diluted, rendering it less effective. Thus, you may spend less money at Spa B and are essentially receiving much less of what you should be getting to achieve your desired results.

If a patient does not know the difference between dilutions, that is understandable. But it is incumbent upon the medical providers to explain to all patients that one clinic's Botox unit is not the same as another clinic's Botox unit. Botox units depend upon how the powdered botulinum-A products are mixed and reconstituted and therefore, it is misleading to give a price per unit of Botox and compare pricing wars.

Now, they are reputable healthcare providers that determine the charge of Botox per unit based upon their knowledge of the patient's treatment goal. However, do not be naive, as medicine is a business, and like many specialties and unscrupulous providers, a disservice can be done not only to the patient but to all healthcare providers if proper disclosure is not presented on how their Botox units are measured. This boils down to trust, and we should all trust our healthcare providers to have our best interest in mind but we all well know that trust must be earned and professionals, these days, whether it's your lawyer, your accountant, your healthcare provider, or your building contractor may not be the best candidate for your hard-earned money. The solution is to pay per area for a job well done.

We are living in a time where we must adhere to that due diligence and understand what we are getting ourselves into and not blindly trust. Most healthcare practitioners that I know are unbelievably trustworthy, however, I will still say every patient needs to walk through that medical office door with the understanding of the problem, ailment, or reason and the treatments necessary to accomplish that task. Do your homework, and Dr. Google is often a great place to start.

The Ethical Practice of Aesthetic Medicine

We all have heard the terms "let the buyer beware" and "the consumer's responsibility is their due diligence" but this takes the blame off of the perpetrator/predator's malicious intent. As a medical professional, I have the obligation, the duty, the responsibility of giving my patients the best possible care with the best possible product, and the best possible understanding of the services to be administered. It is incumbent upon me, and us as practitioners, to make sure that our clients are making the best possible choice by being well informed.

We trust and rightfully so our healthcare providers, the people who sacrificed and spent countless hours learning the science and practice of medicine to care for you. Healthcare providers are there to remove or diminish the ailments that are medically and psychologically damaging to you; that is the main focus of our intended work. However, like many career paths that are chosen with good intentions together with the necessity of earning money to care for ourselves and family, some of us have lost our focus, which saddens me. This is the main reason I chose to consider an alternative to standardized medicine and to practice somewhat independently in medical aesthetics around 2003-2004.

You must always remember that medicine in the United States is a business. It is a legitimate business in which each business has a right to maximize profit, however, there are the wolves in the field just like every other profession. When a wolf captures and kills a sheep to eat, it is neither doing a good thing or bad thing, it is simply living. In the realm of business, patients can get better, patients can be cured, and patients can receive access to good healthcare. However, on the other side of this coin in the realm of this scenario, medicine is a business, and we can be royally screwed by the wolves of this world. Step into a medical spa office with having done your due diligence, having some understanding of the treatment and the cost associated with it and you will leave the medical spa a rejuvenated and well-informed client.

CHAPTER SIX

OVERVIEW OF CURRENT PRODUCTS AND PROCEDURES IN MEDICAL AESTHETICS

Products Competing for Market Share

T oday, the beauty aesthetic market is filled with a plethora of choices for external products used for beautification. However, with medical beauty injectors, we always need to literally go deeper to satisfy the patient's inner desires. Going deeper is diving deep below the skin, below the fatty tissue, and sometimes below the muscle onto the bone to reverse the signs of aging. As we go below the skin, now we get into medical beautification where there are choices, but to a true expert in the field of medical beauty, the choices are very small. Just follow the science, and you will never be swayed away from the truth about what works best and where it works best.

How Botox Works

Botulinum toxin, known to the public as "Botox," is composed of two distinct chains, namely the light chain and the heavy chain, which are connected by a short string. Together, they constitute a single Botox molecule. During the procedure, this Botox molecule, with its heavy and light chains, is injected into specific areas of the face, particularly targeting the lines caused by muscle contractions, such as crow's feet.

Once injected, the heavy chain traverses the surrounding tissue, seeking out nerve cells. It then releases the light chain into the nerve cell. The released light chain serves a crucial role by obstructing the release of chemicals known as acetylcholine(ACH) into the neuro-muscular junction (the space between the nerve and its connection to the muscle. As a result, the muscle fibers are unable to contract. This induced inability to contract leads to either paralysis or relaxation of the muscle strength.

The significance of this mechanism lies in the fact that repeated muscle movements over time contribute to the development of stress lines and cracks on the skin's surface, ultimately resulting in wrinkling of the skin. However, if the muscle is rendered immobile and unable to move, the formation of wrinkles is effectively reduced and prevented.

Relaxing the muscles and removing the contractions that create lines and creases comes down to the practitioner's choice of Botulinum Toxin-A. With the intense marketing of Botulinum toxin brands by big pharma, many have managed to convince the consumer (you) to make these medical choices of medical beauty products on your own.

However, if (you) the consumer does not have adequate medical information to make the choice about what type of Botulinum Toxin-A you would like to have injected in your face, how can you make an informed choice? Many major countries prohibit the advertising of medical drugs and devices to the public for this specific reason.

In 2003, Botox® officially hit the medical world with its Food and Drug Administration (FDA) approval for the removal of lines and wrinkles associated with the orbicularis ocular muscle activity (eye muscles), throwing the beauty industry into a swirl of questions and confusion.

Before Botox®, beauty was only achieved by buying a brand name or top-named skincare brand whether it was removing pimples, removing or adding blush, softening rough skin or clearing up hyperpigmented or blotchy skin or firming up the skin; the products available were your basic drugstore brand topical skincare products or your more expansive doctor recommended expensive brands. Unfortunately, in today's market, we have major pharmaceutical brands competing for the billions of dollars being made from skincare alone, and no two medical aesthetic rejuvenation products are alike.

Botulinum toxin-A products competing for market share starts with the Botox brand FDA approved in 2003 when it was shown to remove lines and wrinkles around the eyes after being used predominantly for overactive muscle twitching of the eyes. When the treating practitioners noticed that the horizontal lines lateral to the lateral cancels known as crow's feet were disappearing and the patients were loving their look after having the strabismus treatment, votes were on their way to becoming a household name.

The Botox™ brand has been around for many years and was slowly followed by another major brand of botulinum toxin-A, which is the Dysport™ brand. Dysport was FDA approved in 2009 as a major competitor to the Botox® brand. In 2009, I was working in medical aesthetics out of a beautiful salon in Queens and had six years of Botox experience. However, I was not comfortable with the delay in the start of the results of removing wrinkles by muscle relaxation.

The reason for my unhappiness with the Botox® brand, after I had done over 1,000 Botox procedures in hundreds of patients was that I always seem to get the same complaint: "When is my Botox going to start?" or "why do I still have lines and wrinkles after one week?" These were the most common complaints I received, and I was unable to remedy my patient's concern other than to explain that it would normally take 7 days to 10 days before the effects of Botox started to work on their faces.

This does not mean the Botox brand is not a good brand, on the contrary, it is an amazing product but for my clientele in New York City, who are used to instant or immediate gratification, I needed a product that kicked in quickly and made the patients smile quicker. In turn, they will return to me in three to four months religiously. and this is exactly what happened. After the introduction of Dysport, these complaints ceased. I no longer fielded calls on complaints of onset of action and reduction of lines and wrinkles so then I was able to concentrate on the other services that I provided when I spoke to the patient after the initial treatment. I was sold on Dysport after a few treatment sessions and from that point, I chose to have a medical spa with only the use of this brand for clients who requested it. I reserved my Botox™ brand for clients who loved it and perceived the best results with it as well.

I proudly consider myself one of the pioneers who embraced Dysport as an excellent choice for my medical spa practice. I knew that the patients who have experienced Dysport treatments would be satisfied with seeing their results in just a few days. This decision propelled my practice to unimaginable heights, surpassing all expectations.

Dysport has been instrumental in the growth of my practice, thanks to its remarkable advantage—an exceptionally fast onset of action. While my peers engaged in pricing conflicts over Botox units, I stood firm in my refusal to conform and rely solely on a brand name. Instead, I opted for multiple brands, which offered my patients a response to their liking and, in my opinion, a superior overall experience. It's truly astonishing to witness the joy on my patients' faces as they beamed with smiles just a few days after receiving beauty injections.

Not Loyal to a Company, But Loyal to Products

From the Greek root of pharmakeia, pharma encompasses herbs or remedies associated with the healing or harmful effects of animals.

And in many cases, it bears true that big pharma can be credited for bringing healing drugs and remedies to medicine governed and operated by non-medical financial enthusiasts. There's no doubt that big for-profit pharmacies are entitled to maximum gains from discoveries and/or manufacturing of drugs and remedies for treatment or cure. No one can tell a company what to make, how to make it, and why they should profit from it in a free market world.

However, this is where ethics and morality come into play, and a company is not a human being or is not an ethical or moral-acting person. A company is an inorganic non-human conceptual entity built or developed for the major purpose of profit. Oftentimes, we feel that the pharmaceutical industry should take care of us or have an obligation to take care of us without understanding that companies are controlled and ruled by individuals or groups with many different philosophies as to the direction of the company and in a free state we all should be allowed to direct or interest and to maximize our profits the best way we know how.

The issue arises when someone else becomes harmed or suffers due to the ambitious pursuits of a company, driven by the desire to gain market share or maximize profit. As individuals who have built companies or even engaged in small side hustles, we understand the objective of generating maximum profit. It's undeniable that if a side hustle begins to generate more income than our primary job, many of us would contemplate leaving our current employment to focus on the profitable venture. In such cases, the side hustle becomes the primary purpose of our entrepreneurial efforts and work.

Therefore, it would be unfair to solely blame big pharma for engaging in similar practices that many of us are capable of and might even consider doing ourselves. It's important to recognize that big pharma is not just a few individuals in a board room; it encompasses all levels of working personnel throughout the industry.

Owners or more accurately, the Board of Directors in big pharma, do not have to be older, well-educated, or experienced businessmen and women; they can be anyone: an Ivy League graduate, a politician, medical personnel/physicians, or just a layperson surviving on their family's inheritance and trust accounts. In the 25 years of practicing medicine, I have owned several corporations and directed care under those corporations for specific reasons first and foremost for profit so I can take care of myself and my family and second, to be able to use my talent and skills to enlighten, treat, and aid in the remedy of the suffering of others whether physical or psychological.

Not Following the Crowd

In my medical beauty practice, I refuse to use products that are not, in my opinion, the very best for the patient's desires. I do not purchase products because they are cheaper so the patient may pay less. In this regard, I will be doing a disservice not only to the patient but also to myself and my practice. I will also inevitably hurt my success and my employees who are depending upon my CEO abilities, my morals, and my ethical standards.

I recently had a client ask me about the swelling that occurs after getting dermal filler treatments. It's a common concern, and my medical explanation to her was that fillers can inherently cause swelling simply by being injected into the face. This is indeed true, as certain dermal fillers have the tendency to cause faster and longer-lasting swelling compared to others. This variation in swelling is primarily influenced by how the filler was formulated and manufactured in the laboratory. Different fillers can inherently create different levels of swelling.

However, it's important to note that the amount of swelling can also vary depending on the specific area of the face where the fillers are placed. When fillers are injected closer to the bone, there may be less noticeable swelling because the structures above, such as muscles, ligaments, fat, and skin, provide resistance to fluid accumulation. On the other hand, if fillers are placed closer to the surface of the skin or just below it, swelling would be more prominent, accompanied by redness and tenderness.

To provide an accurate answer, it's crucial to consider three factors: the choice of filler product by the medical practitioner, the depth of injection chosen by the medical practitioner, and the experience and technique employed by the medical practitioner (the common theme here is becoming clear that the medical provider is the common denominator of poor outcomes). Ultimately, swelling is highly influenced by the skill and decision-making of the medical beauty practitioner and so, the amount of swelling depends on the injector.

While fillers can inherently contribute to swelling, the extent of swelling can be managed and minimized through the expertise of the medical practitioner. It is important for practitioners to carefully consider these factors to ensure optimal outcomes and minimize potential side effects for their patients by understanding that swelling is not always inevitable.

I have a common saying in my practice that every patient who leaves my office should look better than when they came in. Meaning, if there's any swelling, it should be such a minimal amount of swelling that is not noticeable to a stranger on the street. Now, should the medical practitioner be responsible for the swelling if it occurs? Absolutely yes, the medical practitioner is responsible for everything that happens to that patient before they leave the office and after within the duration of that product lasting in the face.

This places a significant responsibility on us as medical practitioners to strive for excellence, take ownership of our actions, and constantly improve upon our abilities to render exceptional patient results. When we acknowledge and accept the blame for the outcomes we contribute to patients, it becomes a catalyst for personal and professional growth. I delivered this speech several years ago to a large audience of medical practitioners, including physicians, surgeons, nurse practitioners, and physician assistants. It may have been the first time many of them had heard the idea that we are accountable for our patients' results.

Just imagine if every surgeon, physician, physician assistant, and nurse practitioner embraced and internalized this concept, using it as a guiding principle in their medical practice. We would undoubtedly achieve far superior outcomes because we would be selective in the products we purchase and use. No single company should monopolize the market or dominate solely based on its brand name. Instead, companies should consistently introduce new and improved products to the market, surpassing previous options or offering superior alternatives.

I personally do not rely on dermal fillers based solely on their brand name. In medicine, we should strive for diversity and healthy competition. By holding companies accountable for producing innovative and effective products, we can avoid using products that yield unpredictable or unfavorable results. It is our duty as medical practitioners to demand and utilize the best available options for the benefit of our patients and the advancement of medical aesthetics.

One challenge when discussing this topic is that in traditional medicine, it is often inappropriate to directly compare drugs. However, in the field of medical aesthetics, if two dermal fillers claim to achieve the same results, it becomes unfair to consumers, patients, and practitioners if we cannot compare these products. I firmly believe that medical aesthetics should not be held to the same standards as standard medical disciplines like cardiology, neurology, orthopedics, or obstetrics and gynecology, etc. The approach, governance, and practice of medical aesthetics must be and is different.

Due to these differences, achieving success in medical aesthetics is not easy. Consequently, many medical practitioners view medical aesthetics as a side hustle rather than their primary focus. When you encounter a dentist, cardiologist, or obstetrician offering Botox treatments in their office, it is essential to question why they feel the need to offer such services. If they are not as successful in their primary specialty, it raises concerns. After all, if they have been practicing for many years and possess various degrees, fellowships, and internships, one would expect them to excel in their chosen field. In my opinion, any medical provider who uses medical aesthetics as only a side hustle while simultaneously struggling in their primary specialty of choice may not be proficient in either specialty.

It is crucial to prioritize specialization and expertise. Attempting to excel in multiple specialties simultaneously may compromise the quality of care provided. Medical aesthetics requires dedicated knowledge, skill, and experience. Therefore, practitioners should focus on honing their expertise in one field before venturing into another.

Story on a Training

In one of my frequent medical teaching sessions, I was tasked with training an established medical office operated by a surgeon and a few of his staff members, notably two nurses, one physician associate, and a medical assistant; This was the medical aesthetic team. Now the surgeon had his operating room in his facility and so was able to do many procedures on site.

Well, being established for well over 15 years, he seemed to be well versed in medical beauty and dermal filler procedures, which always seems to make my job as a trainer more difficult. One of our discussions before I went into the demonstrations was what were the types of fillers he currently uses and why. To my surprise, the practice typically would use only one brand of the dermal filler, and in many instances, they would just grab whatever is on the shelf or whatever the patient requested whether it was a Restylane brand or a Juvéderm brand and start injecting.

This was a huge red flag for me because it told me that the understanding of the different types of fillers had not been well met and my job was to make sure that everyone who trains under me understands that there are vast differences between fillers and even between fillers under the same name brand.

The Science of Fillers

The vast differences in fillers include scientific measures in-vitro (measurements taken within the lab) such as G prime—the ability of the product to resist deformation; the swelling factor—the amount of water retention the product holds onto and drives within; flexibility—the ability for the product to rebound, and last but not least, breakability—the tendency for the product to separate and therefore, migrate.

These few differences are measurements that are taken within the lab to predict what the product would do when injected. However, as I say over and over, what happens in the lab does not necessarily translate to what happens in the human body. Within the human body, there are many other factors that a medical lab cannot replicate because many of the functions that are occurring are happening at once under different dictation and pressure indices and deposited not on a glass Petri dish but either against the bone, within the muscle, within or just below the surface of the skin.

The lab cannot replicate all these biological parameters occurring around the injected fillers. Unfortunately, some offices practice this way typically under one brand and typically based upon what they're found or seen on YouTube or what is trending at the very moment in filler treatments in any particular place such as the lips or the chin.

While these measurements in the lab provide some insights into the product's behavior upon injection, it is crucial to understand that what happens in the lab does not necessarily mirror what happens within the human body. The human body has numerous complex factors at play, which cannot be replicated in a medical laboratory. Functions occur simultaneously under different pressures and conditions, and the product is not deposited on a glass Petri dish but within or against bone, muscle, fat, or just below the skin's surface in the dermis.

Medical Beauty's Requirements: Knowledge and Understanding

To provide the best care for our patients, it is essential to recognize and comprehend the dynamic nature of fillers within the human body. By considering and understanding the unique properties of each filler, we can make informed decisions and achieve optimal outcomes for our patients.

In 2015, I attended a Medical Aesthetic Seminar on dermal fillers and was involved in a think tank on upcoming products for facial rejuvenation. To my surprise, almost all of the injectors had a similar post-injection fullness to the face, many were overfilled and presented the puffy face image that we all know too well now. These injectors have matured in their craft and many no longer have a similar puffy appearance but are actually reveling in their own natural but rejuvenated beauty.

This incident was not a result of inadequate injection techniques but rather stemmed from a lack of comprehension regarding the rheology and scientific properties of Juvéderm Voluma, knowledge which is now well established. Presently, many of these same injectors have significantly improved their facial beauty outcomes. Over the past decade of using Juvéderm Voluma, it has become evident that this product is excellent for specific areas and in precise quantities within the face. As with any profession, injectors have matured in their understanding of both their products and techniques, leading to enhanced results.

However, if those quantities of Voluma are exceeded, then patients will tend to look overfilled, presenting them with a puffy or chubby face. The chubby face that occurs is a response to the product breaking apart and moving upward to the surface of the skin and downward closer to the bone in certain cases this is absolutely a wonderful result but if a patient already has a full face or if too much Juvéderm Voluma is injected into one particular area or if regular touch-ups of additional Juvéderm Voluma are injected several times in or close to the same location, you will see overfilling and stretching of the skin in those areas. Again, this is not a Juvéderm Voluma problem but a practitioner problem.

This can happen with any filler on the market like Restylane brands, however, Juvéderm Voluma has a specific rheologic measure that allows this to occur if the practitioner is not very careful with the quantity of Voluma being injected in any one area.

When I enter a training facility to conduct a medical beauty injectable training, I must first assess the level of experience and know-how within the practice because experience does not equal know-how, and just like every dude ranch and stable that gives horseback riding classes and tours, all the instructors will tell you that most new riders to the establishment always say they know how to ride a horse until it's actually time to ride.

We are all graced with a certain level of ego after performing any task for a considerable amount of time. An ego can be very healthy, and an ego sometimes is necessary, but ego gets in the way of adults learning. Ego is a feeling of self-importance and personal identity amounting to their immediate environment and/or peers. My job as a medical aesthetic trainer is not to crush other's egos but to help them along the way while establishing or maintaining their sense of importance especially if the person being trained is in charge of the medical spa business.

We emphasize the importance of the learning journey. Within the medical field, each of us has likely come across a physician with an excessively inflated ego. Unfortunately, such attitudes can hinder their receptiveness to new insights and learning new skills. For instance, when educating a surgeon about the fundamental and specific scientific aspects of fillers, it becomes crucial to deliver the information in a manner that does not disrupt or undermine their sense of authority and expertise within their medical practice. Our approach is designed to empower them to stay at the forefront of knowledge while incorporating new learnings seamlessly, without implying that they are deficient, thus leaving their ego intact.

How Medical Beauty Dermal Fillers Reach the Market

FDA approval of medical devices such as dermal fillers is based upon the tested location of the face with that particular dermal filler. For example, if a dermal filler is only tested on the chin even though theoretically and practically it could be injected anywhere and sometimes yield better results than if just injected into the chin, its FDA indication/approval can and will only be for the chin.

Therefore, regardless of the location, the dermal filler is best used on the face, let's say the nose, if it was first tested on the lips only, then the FDA indication and approval can only be for the lips. This really means that the pharmaceutical company marketing the dermal filler can only advertise it for the lips otherwise steep fines and penalties may ensue. In order to advertise this lip product for the nose, additional lengthy testing and considerable cost will occur and a duration of testing between 5 and 10 years at times. This, however, is important to ensure the drug/devices are safe and effective in the location and for the purpose being used for.

As an example, there is a product I use in my medical practice to rejuvenate the tear troughs (the area under the lower eyelids that becomes hollow due to genetics and aging) of the face. That product is called Restylane-L, and it is indicated for submucosal implantation for lip augmentation in patients over the age of 21 and also with a specific indication for dermal implantation of the smile lines aka nasolabial folds.

Restylane-L was first FDA-approved in 2005 to treat the smile lines also called nasolabial folds and then later approved for the lips in

2011. Therefore, the original FDA testing for the indication of these two areas had to be done before it could officially be marketed in the United States for these specific areas in the face. Case in point, a filler's FDA indication/approval for use on the face can only be officially marketed for that specific indication.

This brings us to off-label uses of dermal fillers. Off-label uses of a drug such as Botox occur when a drug is prescribed for use other than what the FDA indication/approval is for and outside of what the drug package insert says it should be used for. For many years, from the start of its US debut in medical beauty, up until the late 2010s, Botox was FDA-approved for the glabellar lines, which is the area between the eyebrows called the frown lines.

Although Botox had only this one indication for its cosmetic use, we all were injecting multiple areas of the face including the frontalis muscles for forehead lines, the orbicularis oculi muscles for crow's feet, the nasalis muscles for the bunny lines located on the nose, etc. This was not an illegal act as many drugs are used on areas for reasons other than their indication/approval such as Aspirin, which is approved for pain, fever, cardiovascular disease, whereas off-label uses are for coronary prophylaxis in high-risk diabetics, Semaglutide (Wegovy) is approved for Type-2 diabetes, off-label it is used for weight loss. Gabapentin (Neurontin) is approved for seizures and off-label it is used for pain, alcohol withdrawal, and restless leg syndrome, Sildenifil (Viagra) is approved for erectile dysfunction in men and off-label it is used for female sexual arousal disorder and pulmonary hypertension in children. Morphine is approved for pain in adults and off-label it is used for pain in children.

FDA approval does not mean the best product for the job or area is approved, it only indicates that the product tested in the specific approval site was safe and effective. The best product for the job relies on time and injecting experience. Many dermal filler makers later go onto seek the costly FDA approval for their existing dermal filler in sites already being treated but not indicated so they can make higher profits. Off-label uses for drugs are commonplace and useful to detect the best drug for the job.

There are instances where breaking some of the conventional rules can lead to progress. In the field of medical beauty, where the risk factors are generally low under specific medical guidelines, techniques, and protocols, there is no harm in using a dermal filler in areas that are not FDA-approved. At the level of a medical office, this practice is acceptable. However, at the federal level, pharmaceutical companies are prohibited from advertising their products for uses other than those approved by the FDA. As a result, many dermal fillers are used in areas where they may not be the most suitable option. Additionally, even if a product is FDA-approved for a specific area, the depth in the skin at which it is injected plays a crucial role in achieving the desired results for the patient.

Aftermarket pre-approval of products is a great way to introduce new products for use, but we find that these products need years of maturity in the hands of medical providers to really identify where the products are best suited for based upon the average injection technique. I put emphasis on the average injection technique, which is a very basic beginner-level injecting technique for beginner and intermediate injectors.

During the first 7-8 years of practicing medical beauty, many of my patients experienced a tremendous amount of side effects directly related to poor training. We were not aware of specific or different techniques in administering these drugs and devices, but as a decade passed, we learned so much more in regard to the science of the products but also in regard to the anatomy of the face and the levels and depth of injections that are necessary for our patient's facial features and types of tissue.

One of the major setbacks for beginner injectors is that they may see less than 10 patients a week and just like acting and many other skilled professions, medical beauty injectors require thousands of injecting hours to begin to understand what is truly necessary for a patient's great outcome.

For example, if an injector has been injecting for 10 years at 5 patients per week where each patient procedure is about half an hour, then the injecting hours of the injector equates to approximately 1,300 injecting hours. This is hardly enough injecting hours to begin to have consistency in patient results. Why is this? There are so many types of faces: skin types, tissue texture, shapes, skin tissue thicknesses, tissue ages, tissue laxity and the combinations of these that to get consistency in patient results, takes an extremely long period of time.

As I've always emphasized, it's possible to teach a 12-year-old how to administer Botox and dermal fillers and achieve decent outcomes on an average basis. This is not overly challenging. However, obtaining exceptional results and ensuring patient satisfaction in the range of 95-100% of the time is the true difficulty. This is the standard I aim for when teaching other medical providers. It's not about settling for decent results half the time; it should be about consistently achieving outstanding outcomes 100% of the time. It just takes time.

Achieving consistency in medical beauty procedures hinges upon a thorough grasp of the patient's individual attributes, the targeted tissue, and their specific aesthetic goals. Equally crucial is the ability to skillfully choose the most suitable product for the task. Such decision-making occurs in real-time, during direct conversations with the patient, leaving no room for retreat to a separate area for deliberation. Decisions must be made swiftly, executed with confidence, and without hesitation. Becoming a master injector and a medical beauty expert necessitates ample dedication and practice, as it is a process that takes time for all medical practitioners.

The Side Hustle: Friend or Foe

Medical aesthetics should never be a side hustle. I understand that some practitioners love to be involved in other aspects of medicine while practicing their chosen specialty; however medical beauty deserves a greater amount of respect to accomplish what is necessary for success. If your physician practices hand surgery but also side hustles with cardiology and cardiac surgery, would you be confident in having services performed by them? Medical aesthetics is not different, although, the harm is not as great as dying, and therefore, knowing the risk, people will take the chance if the price is right.

As a medical provider, it is crucial for me to advocate for better drugs on the market, and the same applies to medical beauty practitioners. In the realm of medical beauty, various devices such as fillers and bio-simulators are used to achieve remarkable results when injected into the face. However, it's important to recognize that not all products are created equal, and not all can deliver the same outcomes.

Unfortunately, there are instances where some dermal filler products are known to move/ migrate or shift more than what is considered acceptable. Despite this knowledge, some medical beauty practitioners still choose to use them due to the influence of brand names or patient demand driven by brand advertising. It's important to acknowledge that patients may not possess all the necessary information to make an informed decision, as they may lack comprehensive knowledge of each dermal filler.

If a medical beauty practitioner continues to inject products that are prone to poor outcomes over time, disregarding the inherent risks, they bear responsibility for the patient's poor results. Additionally, if they persist in using subpar drugs/devices instead of seeking the best available fillers, it enables pharmaceutical companies to continue profiting from the sales of these poor dermal filler products, rather than striving to develop better alternatives that would benefit everyone, including the industry.

It is incumbent upon medical beauty providers to invest time in understanding the scientific aspects of the products they use and for the patient to ask questions to confirm the practitioner's knowledge including their technique. Relying solely on the sales representatives of pharmaceutical companies for medical decision-making is absurd. We have witnessed the consequences of such a scenario with the opioid epidemic, where opioids were predominantly prescribed due to the aggressive marketing tactics employed by big pharma.

By staying informed and knowledgeable about what products are available and the science behind these products, medical beauty providers can make more informed decisions and prioritize the well-being of their patients. This approach is crucial to ensure optimal outcomes and avoid potential harm to the patient in the field of medical beauty.

CHAPTER SEVEN

PRESENTING THE DIAMOND TOUCH TECHNIQUE

I n early spring 2010, one of my endearing clients came to visit me for her usual uplifting facial rejuvenation sessions from her favorite injector, me. Vanessa was of Mexican and West Indian descent, and an inspiration, since at such a young age (she was only 35) she had accomplished so much. She was doing very well with her career as a corporate law VP and was recently divorced with two pre-teen children. Vanessa was beautiful, young, intelligent, and full of zest. She had been coming to me for the previous three years for all treatment services that would maintain her youthful appearance and soften or remove the visual signs of aging.

On this occasion, Vanessa sought to replenish her aging cheeks due to some loss of plumpness she once paraded around as her best asset. I gently massaged her anterior cheeks, that area just below her eyes, identifying the specific regions requiring most attention and volume. The goal here was to deliver exactly what she desired and cherished most about herself. None of these treatments matter if she didn't leave my office looking younger. Eagerly anticipating her results before I even started the procedure, I reached for my trusted volume filler at the time and commenced without haste. She was now looking better, and I was now feeling better, smiling, and conversing all the way. My mission was to fulfill her natural beauty and appeal by relentlessly seeking the best techniques with my repertoire of tools.

Now, this was 2010, and the training on aesthetic services using injectables was not as extensive as the teaching sessions I give today. Normally, when a dermal filler product would enter the market for the first time, injectors would have a two-four-hour training session with a pharmaceutical aesthetic trainer. Typically, these trainings are not as in-depth as I would like, due to the time constraints, however, the main focus is on safety and proper usage of the injectable. Most of the techniques typically discussed were done by just about every other practitioner in the same way; the very basic beginner-type injectable techniques that offer the patient decent consistent rejuvenation results in the face.

At this time, I'd been practicing for around seven years, and my clientele was growing steadily due to the techniques I was taught and continued to perfect. However, I was not achieving a high rate of success: 50 to 60% success on patient outcomes and patient satisfaction, therefore I did not have a high patient retention/return. The basic techniques are good for a beginner, but it was not good enough for me, as I had started to establish myself as a serious injector and the feedback on patient experience made me realize I needed to do more extensive anecdotal research and development on existing techniques.

The day Vanessa came to see me for her cheek rejuvenation, she was very excited about the potential results and at the time did not have too many questions about the product or the procedure; she trusted my abilities. So, I gracefully took the dermal filler out of its packaging, carefully laid it onto a clean treatment countertop drape, and started to unwrap the product. I had been using this product for several years to achieve volume in the mid-face. It is also a bio-stimulator, a different kind of filler of sorts, a semi-solid, cohesive injectable implant, whose main ingredient is a synthetic calcium hydroxyapatite particulate suspended in a gel solution of sterile water, glycerin, and sodium carboxymethylcellulose (basically, a gel particle of calcium beads).

I noticed that Vanessa was a bit nervous and apprehensive but was willing to have the procedure done to look her best. After cleaning her face, I started to proceed with her injections to the mid-face, administering one syringe per side of the anterior cheeks. Now, when injecting the cheeks, there is a lot that needs to be considered in terms of the tissue type, the tissue depth, the arteries and veins coursing through the tissue where the bony base lies, along with an understanding of how close to the surface you can inject. Knowing some of these key points is good enough to achieve good results with the basic techniques, but to be an expert, more intricate knowledge is needed. This was an enlightening time, which taught me that I didn't know enough to be an expert yet even after injecting for almost eight years.

After I finished injecting Vanessa's cheeks, I noticed a slight change in the color of her cheeks from rosy-red, which occurs most procedures, to a more grayish hue, pale, and cool. I had no idea what was in store for me for the next several months. Vanessa developed a compressive occlusion from the quantity of product injected within the specific location, likely abutting her angular artery and presenting with an avascular sequelae. This is a very big deal and one of the sphincter's alerts that we as injectors hear about. Possible occlusions can lead to blindness at worst, permanent necrotic scarred tissue, or in the least, a few months of red and angry-looking tissue and skin.

Post-injection occlusions of the face can be scary for both the patient and the medical provider. Anastomosis refers to the merging of two or more blood vessels, forming a unified path. It is possible for an occlusion, caused by dermal fillers, to obstruct the flow of blood through this anastomosis from the lower face to the vessels behind the eyes causing vision impairment, temporary blindness, and or permanent blindness. Also, when the filler product binds with water and expands, it intensifies the blockage, preventing the supply of oxygen and nutrients to the tissue beyond that particular occluded vessel. Therefore, it is crucial to observe any changes in color within the treated area immediately after the procedure, as this may indicate an impending and serious mechanical flow issue known as filler embolism or vascular occlusion.

It's easy to get some understanding of vascular occlusions when you read or listen to discussions in a forum, event, or classroom. But when you come across it for the first time in person, your mind goes blank because you know there could be blindness, tissue damage, and expensive legal problems can arise from it. The worst nightmare for any medical aesthetic injector is occlusions or blockages of arteries or veins caused by dermal fillers or bio-stimulators like Radiesse™ or Sculptra™. That's exactly what happened to me and my patient on that unfortunate night. Vanessa had no idea how serious it was, but I did. As I started perspiring suddenly and feeling extremely worried, I had to keep my cool and be confident so that Vanessa wouldn't freak out. This wasn't the first time it happened to me either, Vanessa was my third occlusion case, and there had to be a reason why. In medicine, it's all about numbers, so back to the drawing board.

One course of action would have been to send Vanessa to the emergency department for observation and care, however, hospital emergency medical personnel (physicians, nurses, PAs, etc.) do not have a clue about medical beauty products, treatments, and adverse events. Therefore, sending Vanessa to the hospital would have yielded no additional treatment than I could have offered her, but one thing it would have given her would have been excessive cost and irrelevant testing. Knowing this, I proceeded to give her dermal care typically reserved for wound patients.

About the numbers, the more treatments you perform, the more possible adverse outcomes you'll encounter, which means a higher chance of adverse reactions and serious negative outcomes. For instance, if you only inject five people a week, it's unlikely that you'll encounter any major issues because the number of injections performed is too low. But if you're injecting 75-100 people a week, you're bound to come across a lot more problems. And that was exactly my case. I faced way more issues than the average injector at the time because my injection volume was sky high. I believe I was considered one of the top five injectors in several neighboring counties, if not the entire Queens area, apart from one or two dermatology/surgical medical spas.

Putting an End to Uncertainty and Madness

When Vanessa became my third case of vascular occlusion, I knew I had to do something to prevent these potential disasters from happening again. I spent weeks pondering this issue, trying to wrap my mind around what was going on and searching for a better alternative to common side effects of medical beauty treatments, if one existed. At that point, my understanding of injecting was simply pushing the needle through the skin to a certain depth and delivering the drug or medical device, like dermal fillers, into the body.

It was during this time that I realized the importance of mastering the instrument in my hand, which eventually led me to question the entire injecting process and create a different method of injecting called Diamond Touch Technique.® What were all the steps involved? What instruments or products were used in each of these steps that ultimately determined the outcome for the patient? These were some of the questions that needed to be answered, and it was the beginning of a complete overhaul of my injection technique and approach.

The Syringe-Needle Device

The first case is the syringe-needle device. If the problem of vascular occlusion was occurring because of the syringe needle and every injector is using the same syringe needle, then everyone may be having the same problem, over time, as I was encountering. Also, if I was being trained the same as everyone else with the same syringe-needle, then it meant that everyone else had to have been going through the same scenarios as me and therefore, something had to be changed or be modified. Following the injection instructions of everyone meant that I was average, and my techniques were then average, which lead to average results and average patient satisfaction. Today, we cannot change the syringe-needle device yet since most used syringe-needle devices are similar, and changes would require huge amounts of money, testing, and marketing for a better syringe-needle to hit the market. Therefore, the syringe-needle became a constant in this equation.

The ATP of Medical Beauty Injections

Three things come together to create a superb patient outcome. Anatomy, technique, and Product (or what I call the ATP process). Together, these form my core powerhouse for patient satisfaction outcomes, so I knew I had to research each component and look for variables that would lead to higher patient satisfaction.

In just a matter of days, Vanessa's left cheek, just below her left eye, started to display an angry red hue, eventually developing into an ulcerated flesh wound. Such a distressing outcome is the last thing any injector wishes to witness, as it brings forth significant issues like potential disfigurement for the patient and the looming threat of legal repercussions if not handled appropriately.

At that time, no emergency medical department in any hospital was familiar with injectable products, their possible complications, or how to address such problems. This placed the entire responsibility on me to ensure Vanessa's face healed properly. The situation was an immense source of embarrassment for both Vanessa and I. Vanessa, a valued long-term patient and a beautiful young woman, entrusted me with her care, and I found myself facing the possibility of permanently harming her face.

This incident kept me up at night since the facial tissue wound, if not treated well, could form a very ugly facial scar. Bear in mind, there was no one there to help me at that time. Medical beauty procedures were still seen as elitist and hyper-vain, and any problems occurring because of it was considered the patient's fault, and the medical provider could lose or have his or her license suspended. This was unfair. Medical beauty was in its infancy then and today medical beauty is in its adolescence now. We have learned so much but there's still so much left to learn.

I could not continue practicing with the same techniques that I had learned from the previous injectors, the podium speakers, and the stage presenters. I had to find out what the circumstances were that make vascular occlusions more probable and how I could prevent this problem in the future. Therefore, I had to find a way to update my injectable practices to safeguard my career and livelihood.

In 2010, after Vanessa's experience with me, I immersed myself in understanding all of the scientific components of fillers and bio-stimulators and also investigated the standard techniques compared to possible new techniques: the when, why, where, and the how of all the injectable products from Botox to bio-stimulators. It was very interesting to find out that most of the information I needed was not accessible and unattainable from any of my usual sources, so I had to dive into European, Asian, and South American literature to get more input on the products and procedures. I came to find out that most of the problems occur from the techniques used in administering the medical beauty products, therefore originating with the practicing provider, i.e., most of the problems occur from the injectors themselves and not the injectable products. These injectable products are just tools and like tools, choosing the wrong filler for the job and injecting in a less-than-effective technique will always lead to a higher incidence of adverse events like vascular occlusions.

Negating the Blame

If your carpenter fixes your roof and does a horrible job and ruins your roof, you don't blame the hammer, the nails or the material used, you blame the carpenter. But as I pointed out earlier, the difference between standard medicine and medical beauty is that standard medicine finds it easy to blame the product-devices, to blame the diseases; high blood pressure, to blame the drugs; diabetic drugs, and to blame the non-steroidal anti-inflammatory (NSAIDs) for the stomach ulcers. This should not occur because the blame lies with the practitioner who prescribed the drugs and who injects the medical beauty products. The fault lies with us, and we must take action and accept accountability to address the issues by understanding what we did to facilitate the poor results. This is why I founded Diamond Touch Technique.®

The Enthusiast for the Avant-Garde: Starting Over

One of the first things I wanted to reconstruct was my understanding of human facial anatomy. Medical beauty is a relatively new area of interest within medicine and closely linked to dermatology more so than cosmetic surgery. It's an entirely new field of expertise or subspecialty that has emerged to treat the patient physically without understanding its true psychological nature. The problem was that most medical textbooks on facial anatomy before 2010 didn't truly capture all the intricacies and latest knowledge and updates we have today on facial anatomy because of the newness of medical beauty.

As a result, the training we received on facial anatomy wasn't enough to make us experts in precision facial medical beauty. The human face is made up of various components: fat pads, muscles with their nerve supply, specific muscle origins and attachments, functional expressions, fascia and ligamentous structures, and how the facial bones interact with this anatomy. Facial plastic surgery, which preceded medical beauty injections but didn't influence its growth, did a great job of understanding and mapping gross facial anatomy. However, it can be seen as a more broad, big-picture approach to facial rejuvenation. On the other hand, medical beauty took a more detailed and fine-tuned approach to overall facial anatomical aging.

For example, if you are having your kitchen redone, typically the contractor who is working on the flooring is not the same individual that does the finishing touches to the walls and overall finish of the kitchen. Can the general contractor do all? Of course, yes. However, like all other crafts, one person cannot be an expert in all things. Meaning that the general contractor cannot be as good as the highly specialized individual who only does the finishing touches to kitchens (cabinets, mounting, sheetrock, sanding, and finished painting) eight hours a day every working day. Medical beauty injectors are like no other craftsmen in the field of medicine; however, this does not take away from the other medical craftsmanship.

Medical beauty is the highly specialized finishing touch to fine-tuned facial beauty. While facial plastic surgery will address the larger macro-manipulation of the face, medical beauty will address the smaller intricate micro-manipulation consisting of harmony between angles and curves necessary for a beautiful and youthful face. This is why many patients undergoing full plastic surgery for a facelift never seem to look great after the surgery unless dermal fillers and botulinum toxin are also employed for an overall comprehensive outcome.

Put another way, post-surgical facelifts require the administration of medical beauty injectables to achieve a beautiful final result. This point is undeniable with a resounding aha moment. It will also explain why medical beauty is the fastest-growing medical industry in the entire world and why many physicians and practitioners practicing standard medicine outside the field of medical beauty are looking to medical beauty as a lucrative option to transition into as side hustles.

Back to the evolution of the Diamond touch technique. First, my job was to traverse the most recent medical literature on facial anatomy which was not in standard medical textbooks. Most of this information was still found online through multiple sources and had to be pieced together to form a full picture of facial anatomy. This was my very first step to understanding the anatomy of the human face and its intricacies to allow a precise working knowledge of facial anatomy for consistent and optimal results.

Second, in the ATP of medical beauty and by far the biggest change necessary, was overhauling the entire medical beauty injection techniques for Botulinum toxin, dermal fillers, and bio-stimulators. This was by far no easy task since there was no precedent to what I was doing. There were a handful of mix and match techniques intertwined with basic techniques, and it was a free-for-all at this point. The challenge was to break down the different types of techniques, and show what works, what doesn't work, and what is integral to the success of consistent positive outcomes for patients.

Some basic techniques in the medical beauty field are single boluses, multiple repeating boluses, fanning, cross-hatching, and the super popular retrograde threading technique. These are the fundamentals that I rarely use or incorporate into any of my treatments. Apart from studying and understanding these techniques on paper, it was also my responsibility to gather feedback from my recurring patients. I wanted to know what worked, what didn't work, what gave temporary results, what gave long-lasting results, and what was least traumatic for the patient's face. I spent countless nights analyzing patient charts, comparing before and after pictures, and considering treatment options against the actual treatment provided.

Now, here's the thing: thanks to my high patient retention rate, I got to witness everything firsthand. This was my ever-so-needed anecdotal evidence. I made it a point to see all my patients two weeks after their injections, which was not an easy task. It was exhausting, tedious, and overwhelming. For example, let's say I saw 20 patients on a Wednesday, and then two weeks later, I had to see those same 20 patients plus another set of 15-20 new treating patients. It made for a seriously busy day. But if you want to be better than everyone else, you can't just do what everyone else is doing. That's the mantra I always repeat to my interns and trainees: strive to be better with every patient treatment, don't settle for the status quo, and rely on your anecdotal evidence with documentation when you can.

The third and final consideration in the ATP of medical beauty is product selection. The drug companies would gladly want you to believe that one or a few of their products does everything. The reality is each product conforms to a certain set of characteristics that limit how much they can do. For example, we have some soft fillers that cannot do what firmer fillers would do and vice versa. If I am looking for a high projection on the patient's boney cheeks, I cannot use a soft low G-prime product. I must use a firmer higher G-prime product. On this note, let's look at G-prime as one of the main scientific numbers that contribute to what a product does in the face. G-prime or G is a value given to a product based upon its resistance to applied external forces and movement, i.e., what it does under force, pressure, and shearing stress.

One of my classic and favorite examples is the analogy that explains what G-prime is. If you take a heaping spoon of peanut butter and you stack that spoon of peanut butter on a countertop then next to that peanut butter you take a heaping spoon of strawberry jam and stack that jam on the same counter next to the peanut butter and return in 24 to 48 hours, you will have a stack of peanut butter looking at exactly as you placed it standing tall and firm versus the flattened, spread-out strawberry jam.

This is a perfect example of G-prime. The higher the G-prime, the higher the resistance to deformation/damage/change or movement of the product. And therefore, peanut butter has a higher G-prime number than strawberry jam, which has a very low G-prime. Dermal fillers use these same values where some dermal fillers have the strength of peanut butter while other dermal fillers lack strength and spread outward like strawberry jam.

Now the lowest G-prime would be considered water and the highest G-prime would be considered a rock, both are substances that have internal motion (yes, even rocks have internal movement). However, the rock can stand without deformation/change for centuries unless enough force is applied to it to either break, smash or scatter it. Then, there is the water with the absolute lowest G-prime that will conform to any shape or size with a minimal amount of outside pressure/force, mostly just gravity. This analogy has helped me in explaining G-prime to my interns and my trainees.

All dermal fillers on the market have a G-prime value. This G-prime value helps us understand what the dermal filler product will and will not do, can and cannot do. In standard medicine, many treatment providers depend upon pharmaceutical representatives for information on new products entering the market. This should not be the only resource the medical beauty injector uses.

In medical beauty, we tend to do the same thing though, we rely on pharmaceutical representatives to give us information on the newest dermal fillers or the existing dermal fillers and what their potential properties will do in the face. This again should be minimized to avoid multiple different drug representatives inadvertently giving contrary information. The final determination of the dermal product's abilities should be ascertained by the medical beauty injector with whom the patients will consult with. There should be selective unbiased sources that can give this information readily to all practitioners, thereby allowing the best products to remain ahead of the game.

My years in orthopedic medicine and surgery taught me that medical beauty injectors need to do their own research on drugs and medical devices such as dermal fillers before introducing them to patients. At the time of the opioid epidemic and the thirst for opioid prescriptions, we had many pharmaceutical representatives pushing codeine and codeine-like drugs to our post-surgical patients through medical practitioners such as surgeons, PAs, and nurses. We now know that was a tremendous mistake and many people either died or became addicted, ruining not only their lives but the lives of the loved ones around them.

As a medical professional, my top priority is to "do no harm" physically, mentally, or financially to my patients. That's why, whether I see them again in a few weeks or never see them again, I always keep their well-being in mind. I firmly believe that we should never introduce any remedies, drugs, or devices that could potentially harm the patient in the future; this is one reason I am against the continued use of silicone microdroplet injections in patients' faces.

We have a responsibility and are legally accountable for the outcomes of our actions and the patient's results. Medical ethics is something I carry with me wherever I go, and one of its core principles is to prioritize the safety and welfare of the patient. If that means opting for a product that may not last as long but poses less risk, rather than using a product that offers longer-lasting results but could potentially cause harm, the safer option will always be the right option.

Product selection is a major component of overall patient satisfaction. No two products are alike, and no two products do the same job in the face. Besides G-prime, there are quite a few other scientific values that are necessary for the provider to understand before they can choose the right product for their patient.

Next, concerning the products: does the dermal filler add to the problem of potentially adverse events and poor outcomes? If it is indeed the case that the product may have been inadequate to yield good results, then we need to find the source of the problem within that product. However, if the product is not known to be associated with a high incidence of poor outcomes, then the technique that was used with that specific product must be investigated, modified or changed entirely.

In the case of Vanessa's adverse event, vascular compromise, my conclusion led me to believe that the technique that was used may have been the primary causative variable leading to the ischemia that developed that lead to tissue damage. Luckily, having a reasonable understanding of skincare allowed me to resolve all of Vanessa's vascular compressive episodes with zero noticeable after effects such as scarring or disfigurement.

Being proactive, if my conclusion was that my technique was inadequate thus leading to high incidences of adverse events, then I must change my injection technique. This was my epiphany. And so, Diamond Touch Technique was born out of necessity. Necessity is the mother of invention after all.

The Diamond Touch Technique

The significance of Diamond Touch Technique has two key aspects: First, the uniqueness of each diamond gem crafted to perfection resembles and mirrors our unique features surprisingly well, and second, the touch of the practitioner's hand when administering treatment plays a vital role in achieving beauty according to your desires. Let's first dive into the second half of the technique, which is the "Touch" portion of the Diamond Touch Technique.

This was the answer to many of my previous injecting issues pre-2010 with patient outcomes that stemmed from the basic pharmaceutical-guided training that I received before 2010. Pharmaceutical-guided training consisted of the basic techniques for beginner and intermediate injectors, however, the techniques being taught and used like any new procedure is a set of protocols good enough for the average injector and will render reasonable results. Modifying the basic techniques to a more advanced option to suit a larger scale clientele base and client demand was a game-changer.

As medical beauty injectors advance in their career, the basic techniques start to become somewhat inadequate with shortcomings leading to poor patient outcomes. Some of these shortcomings include: continued excessive side effects, an inherent loss of confidence with the patient, staff members, and the injectors themselves. Advanced and innovative injecting techniques are necessary for growth within the craft of this industry, limiting adverse events and bad outcomes. As medical beauty experts, we should have a high degree of confidence that the outcome and the patient's satisfaction will be good with every treatment; this is predictability.

The Diamond Touch Technique was founded to relieve the patient's unnecessary side effects and relieve the medical spa/injector/myself of potential legal and financial liability. In turn, the utmost benefit is relieving the client of traumatic/physical and psychological harm such as embarrassment from others, embarrassment toward themselves, judgment from family, friends, and strangers, as well as psychological scarring—this is the harm allotted to patients when the technique and product selection is not well determined.

When I hear Diamond Touch Techniquem, I think of no bruises, no redness, virtually no excessive pain, and no facial distortion in 100 percent of clients that I touch with the "Diamond Touch." Taking the time to create the Diamond Touch Technique was one of the most productive and effective measures I have taken in my entire medical career. Upon execution of this technique, I was able to drastically reduce the number of patient complications and issues that occurred. While the Diamond Touch Technique was not the easiest procedure to learn, neither is making a Stradivarius.

I am sure that Antonio Stradivari did not get it right the first time and spent thousands of labored hours to get the right pitch, tone, and feel of the string instrument he made most popular, known as the Stradivarius violin. In a well-known 2008 book titled "Outliers" a memorable quote was made famous by its author, Malcolm Gladwell who said, "10,000 hours is the magic number for greatness." Gladwell is still alive and writing and what he meant was that to be considered a highly specialized and expert craftsman, you must practice for at least 10,000 hours to become an expert and gain the respect or at least the acknowledgment of your peers.

This translates to approximately 20,000 medical aesthetic procedures. For example, a typical botulinum toxin treatment may take 20 to 30 minutes and a typical dermal filler treatment may take 30 minutes totaling one hour, so for a sum of 10,000 hours, it would take you 20,000 procedures of botulinum toxin and dermal filler injections. Achieving this takes well over 10 years since many injectors see less than 25 patients a week.

It is safe to say that I blew past these 10,000 hours a very long time ago due to my high-volume injecting practice in New York City, and I do consider myself an expert but reluctantly so. Why reluctantly? Because there are so many nuances to the treatment that must be learned. Medical beauty is still new and in its young stage, true experts are hard to come by. Unfortunately, most injectors paint themselves as advanced or experts after only a few years of injecting a handful of patients a week. And then there are the few who have been injecting for many years and still would not consider themselves advanced or experts but do an amazing job; those are the true giants of the industry.

Between cosmetic surgery and medical beauty, the scalpel and the syringe-needle are the most frequently used instruments. Both these devices carry their weight in gold, and they become the extension of the practitioner's fingers. It takes years to finesse the use of a scalpel and every surgeon, every successful surgeon must be commended. However, it also takes several years to understand the intricacies of the hypodermic needle; its use goes far beyond simple sticks and understanding the hypodermic needle's secrets allows me to understand what I am doing as I place that needle below the surface of my patient's skin.

The needle tip naturally possesses a 4-sided bevel and an angle, enabling them to cut and slice through tissue with ease. This is great for vaccinations or deep quick needle puncture medication administration but not for medical beauty detailing of the face. Consequently, there is a need to reimagine and reinvent the hypodermic needle for use exclusively in medical beauty, and I hope to contribute to that effort with the available time and resources it needs. When inserting the hypodermic needle into the tissue, the angled tip causes it to deviate from a straight path. Depending on the side of the needle's opening, known as the bevel, the product can be delivered to different locations inadvertently.

Sometimes, we want the bevel of the needle to face the skin surface, while other times we want it to face away from the skin surface.

In certain instances, we want the bevel to face the fat pads, while in others, we want it to face away from the fat pads. Each specific procedure determines whether we desire the bevel to face the tissue, the skin surface, or the opposite direction, but always at some angle or another.

Understanding the use of the needle helps us avoid the common mistakes that cause bruising, redness, swelling, and pain. Typically, these are called normal side effects of the injecting needle; nonetheless, they can be avoided. No one leaves my office swollen, bruised, red, or in pain. This is super convenient for clients who are on the go in and out of our offices during break, lunchtime, or in transit between leaving the office and heading home. It is difficult to comprehend the overwhelming effect of having to return home from a medical spa visit with a reddened face, swelling, and pain from medical beauty injections plus having to explain and justify to anyone critiquing the reason for your visit. With Diamond Touch Technique, this is a thing of the past. Every client should leave looking better than they came in.

THE LUST FOR MEDICAL BEAUTY

DISCOVERING THE PERFECT INJECTOR

Difference Between a Master of Mind and a Practitioner

Several years ago, I was blessed to have the means and time to completely remodel our home. This was such an important time for my family, and I set about to locate the best contractor for the project. The decision to overhaul the house came with a plethora of jobs to be completed from local permits to everything that needed to be worked on from the roof that needed replacing to extensive ceiling repair, and a complete gut of the upper floor, ground floor, flooring, windows in need of an upgrade, and finally landscaping around the perimeter of the house. (It kind of reminded me of a complete mommy make-over.)

Since practicing orthopedic medicine for several years, I have met many professionals in all walks of life and careers. Some were building and construction contractors and one who became a friend by the name of Matthew agreed to renovate for me. Mathew came to the house one early morning ready to give me his estimate for the necessary jobs and ended up proposing to work on the roof, and perform general carpentry, as well work on the electrical, flooring, plumbing, and landscaping. This was great, since it was a one-stop shopping experience and therefore, I didn't have to go hunting for valuable experts for each job. I felt reassured that this house remodel would go off without a hitch but sadly, without knowing that it rarely ever happens.

Fast forward two months into the various home renovation jobs and everything was still creeping along slowly. I later found out that Matthew's expertise was only carpentry, and it was necessary for him to subcontract out the rest of the key projects, especially when tackling the bathrooms and the kitchen. He seemed to be able to do it all, but unfortunately, he was doing it all but not doing it well! Matthew appeared to be an expert who seemed to have a keen understanding of building projects and a keen sense of knowing what the customer needed. He was not great at any one task and so he listed himself as a general contractor where he would subcontract many aspects of the building processes to other experts.

General contractors seem like well-rounded people, but when it comes to actually doing a great job that's worth the customer's hard-earned money, it's a different story. Similarly, in medicine, you don't see practitioners who are knowledgeable and well versed in one specialty like obstetrics and gynecology try to practice another specialty like pediatrics; they can't possibly do as good a job as specializing in one specialty. That's where the problem lies in medical beauty. While Matthew did a decent job on some projects, overall, he didn't do a great job in the overall work.

The medical field tends to view medical beauty as a mere add-on for making extra money. Medical beauty is seen as something simple where you can charge cash and make a significant profit within an already existing practice specialty. However, I believe that medical beauty is not just an add-on to other specialties like surgery or dermatology; it's a specialty that requires dedication and extensive knowledge (facial anatomy, product rheology, facial morphology, procedural techniques, etc.) in order to excel at it.

The Paradox of Knowledge

The more knowledge you attain, the more knowledge is unattained. A doctorate degree or Ph.D. can take up to eight years to achieve. The more PhDs achieved relates to the amount of time lost from gaining many other facets of knowledge due to the immense amount of time necessary to attain a Ph.D. Similarly, the more time spent to be highly specialized and learn one specific topic, the more time is lost gaining wider views of other topics. This does not mean it is not wise to reach for higher specific knowledge; what this means is we should not administer an all-knowing or worldly status to a highly specialized individual. Therefore, we welcome artificial intelligence and its promises if used virtuously.

This does not mean that a practitioner cannot cover more than one specialty. However, would you like your pediatrician to surgically operate on you or your general practitioner to do your breast implants? I am certainly not saying that one practitioner should not venture out of their chosen board-certified specialty to practice another specialty. If the dedication to the knowledge and craft of that specialty is met, a practitioner can be a specialist in more than one area.

The problem here is that medical beauty does not have a specific credentialing organization or set of requirements to perform these intricate beauty treatment tasks, and for this, the smell of quick money and high profits excites everyone to dive into medical beauty, which is a designer specialty that does more than design the face to a patient's whims and wants. Medical beauty has a wide and far-reaching benefit to all who receive a good result. The psychological impact on everyone touched by botulinum injections is just incredible. No longer is medical beauty relegated to surgeons with price tags beyond belief. With a good result, smiles and elation is what we observe when medical beauty is used appropriately, in good judgment, and with the patient's best interest in mind.

People tend to not only radiate beauty, but also treat others around them better when they themselves look better or feel good about themselves. When you look good, you feel good. When you look and feel better it is also likely that negative comments or actions against you are not absorbed as much. Looking better is in the hands of the injector and the expectations of the patient.

Your general contractor is incapable of creating a beautiful new bathroom or kitchen without the help of an expert specifically trained in either area and therefore should not be the ones to actually do the work. Your dentist cannot render as good a result as the injector treating patients every day, eight hours a day. It truly takes an incredible amount of time and practice to perfect the art of facial designing and redesigning. Now, there are many surgeons and non-surgical practitioners with extensive knowledge to perform medical aesthetics, but it is undeniable that the practitioner who only immerses themselves in medical beauty injections 8+ hours a day, 5 days a week is going to be an exceptional craftsman.

Evaluating the Reliability of Credentials: Are We Safe?

I accompanied a friend to the urologist because she was experiencing discomfort in her back suddenly after a night out with some friends. I suspected it was kidney stones based on the presentation of her complaints and her sudden debilitating pain with nausea and vomiting. While waiting in the urologist's waiting room, I noticed an entire wall of framed diplomas and certifications. Initially, seeing these diplomas and certifications had a reassuring effect on me but as I looked closer, I noticed all the diplomas and certifications were acquired 10-20 years ago and the most recent certification was several years back.

Now, I was struck with a peculiar feeling of uncertainty. I know the reason for the grand display of the diplomas and certifications, but it sends a different message when the dates are over a decade old. Does this mean that the doctor did not further his education or procedural methods? The realization of this struck me as odd and forced me to reevaluate what I do in my medical office in reference to displaying my certifications. I currently do not display certifications; however, I do list all of my credentialing activities including speaking events on advanced medical aesthetic topics, cadaver instruction that I am proud to be a part of, and my continuing medical education, which is a mandatory activity every two years.

Therefore, outdated framed credentialing did the opposite of instilling confidence since any diploma or credential only speaks of the abilities of the medical provider at that time of the granted certification. People—and medical providers are people—change in their physical ability and their mental acuity levels from year to year. I would have been more comfortable seeing an updated, within the past two years, certification on the wall of displayed certifications.

Regarding medical beauty, this again is a very new specialty, therefore educational data, products, and procedures have evolved considerably making any training in medical beauty over a decade ago obsolete and simply inadequate for today's standards. Don't display old diplomas to garner confidence; show the client what you are doing to remain on top of the knowledge base necessary for them to trust your abilities.

Due Diligence, Trust, and Medical Care

In all medical specialties, the patient is obligated to do their due diligence, as the homework in researching the medical provider is key in the preparation for optimal care of themselves or loved ones. It's easier to trust in faith than to do the research necessary on the individual treating us. Sometimes, we all have a tendency to blindly trust medical personnel without question, even myself, I was guilty of this. Unfortunately, this can sometimes result in mistakes, substandard care, and even loss of lives (indirectly due to psychological harm) when we fail to properly ensure that our healthcare provider (such as a doctor, physician assistant, or nurse) is well-informed and up-to-date in their area of expertise, specifically in the field of medical aesthetics. Trust your medical practitioner, but do not "blindly" trust your medical practitioner.

Diplomas merely certify that a practitioner attained the knowledge necessary to practice medicine or surgery at that time of graduation. A diploma certainly does not say that for the next 10 years, this individual will be great at their medical career. Nothing guarantees optimal service, however certifications or acknowledgments of present or recent practices help to confirm adequacies in the medical care you receive. After all, medical aesthetics is still considered medical care.

Current education is so important to the well-being of the patient that if the injecting practitioner is behind in the most recent evidence-based and procedural-based knowledge, then patient harm can occurs. I will argue that there is a tremendous amount of psychological harm done to patients every day in the medical world. The common notion is that Botox doesn't kill or create any real physical harm, but that is absolutely incorrect.

A substantial amount of psychological harm, financial harm, and many times, unseen physical harm, which by the way is seldom reported out of embarrassment by the patient, occurs more than we think. The medical literature on facial anatomy was grossly outdated up to 10 years ago, and now the new medical literature on facial anatomy is catching up to the fast pace of medical aesthetics; therefore any practitioner not up to date on the current literature can do severe harm to their patients even if that harm is not being reported. Many of my new consultation patient complaints are of their previous medical beauty treatments due to poor results.

Back to the story of the diploma-patterned wall. In the corner of the waiting room there was a small table with a cornucopia of medical beauty pamphlets and brochures being offered for the patient's convenience. My first thought was if a practitioner is practicing for over 10 years in any specialty, then after 10 years, they should be inundated with a substantial patient volume rendering them unable to do or practice any other specialty outside of their board-certified specialty. I practiced orthopedics for 10 years early in my career and by year five, I did not have any available time to touch any other specialty just by the volume of patients returning due to the provision of good services.

Any medical practitioner looking to change specialties and who whole-heartedly enters medical beauty with the passion and determination to be great at practicing medical aesthetics is commendable. However, treating medical aesthetics as a side hustle brings many doubts about the adequacy of their own chosen specialty and begs the question as to why the multi-specialty practitioner is not doing well enough to be successful in their own chosen specialty. Medicine should never be seen as a side hustle; this is an insult to all specialties that deserve immense dedication and is an insult to the patient's trust.

Plastic and cosmetic surgeons are capable of providing excellent care to the patient with an extensive background in anatomy and facial architecture. However, the use of a needle is certainly different from the use of a scalpel. Some surgeons demonstrate great results both in the needlework of medical beauty and the scalpel work of reconstruction but more often than not, I hear patients touting different levels of care and treatment when it comes to medical beauty from other injectors outside of surgical practices.

Medical beauty injectables is an excellent adjunct to the practice of plastic and cosmetic surgery but only if the surgical practice has a dedicated injector to oversee and treat the separate medical beauty injection aspect of the patient's beauty care. Many surgeons currently do just that and this is commendable and responsible for them not to try to take on all surgical and injectable services together by themselves while being inundated with their own surgical patients.

This is by no means an attack on facial plastics or cosmetic surgery but an attempt to enlighten readers that great care can come from multiple medical-oriented disciplines and personnel. No individual credential shall dominate or monopolize a specialty. That is like stating that only orthopedic surgeons are capable of treating musculoskeletal problems and diseases and chiropractors, acupuncturists and alternative specialties have no place in musculoskeletal care.

This very sentiment was maintained for many years before chiropractors, acupuncturists, and alternative specialties like reiki, acupressure, movement specialists, and so on were accepted as being specialists who could create positive patient outcomes in musculoskeletal care although it took a considerable amount of time. The same holds true for Doctors or Osteopathy (DOs) who had a difficult time breaking into all aspects of medicine and being seen as equal to the status of the MD.

When it comes to seeking medical care, the responsibility falls on the patient to diligently find the best healthcare professional available for them. Unfortunately, relying on other medical personnel working within the same medical practice to offer you advice on the proficiency of the treating staff in that medical practice is neither ideal nor logical. It would be more advantageous to have a reliable review system in place for all practitioners, similar to Google Reviews, without the fear of patients being subjected to legal action.

This review system currently occurs on a large scale, but only with medical beauty so why is that? This should be the case for all medical disciplines, after all, every one of us including all doctors, PAs, and nurses will require medical and surgical care at some point, and we will be at the hands of any medical practitioner without knowing their true abilities to care for us with the utmost respect and dedication to their specialty.

Implementing a system like Google Reviews for all disciplines of medicine faces challenges including the potential for inaccurate patient complaints, personal grudges, and biased algorithms designed with hidden agendas favoring higher-paying practitioners. In the current landscape, a combination of verbal referrals and Google Reviews appears to be the most effective means of evaluating the competence of a specific medical beauty practitioner. It is widely acknowledged that relying solely on magazine article ads or websites proclaiming a practitioner as a top doc or best of the best is not the wisest approach to judge competency.

Navigating the Beauty Maze: Differentiating Talent

Everyone has a specific God-given talent whether discovered or not. We all have our strengths and weaknesses that dictate where our comforts lie and that may lead to our chosen final career destination. There are three fundamental types of professional aptitudes with innate abilities to accomplish tasks in their chosen professions like medical beauty.

1- THE SPATIALLY INTELLIGENT: Ones who excel with their mental abilities predominantly such as individuals who thrive in a spatial element of cognitive mapping, where concepts and solutions are derived from their thoughts—scientists, computer programmers, writers, anyone with a Ph.D. or doctorate, influencers, CEOs, CFOs, COOs, financial specialists, etc. Basically, anyone who does not need to work with their hands predominantly to accomplish tasks well. Someone who enjoys spatial thinking to solve problems using algorithmic concepts. These are the smart individuals who could not use a screwdriver if their life depended upon it, but they can do your taxes, explain the intricacies of the universe, and explain why your life may or may not matter.

2- THE PHYSICALLY INTELLIGENT: Ones who excel with physical abilities predominantly such as individuals who thrive in a more geometrical space, where physical attributes are the focus to build upon. These are the contractors (carpenters, masonry, plumbers, electricians), athletes, surgeons, and injectors. The professionals that build, repair, or modify structurally find a sense of joy in a trance-like state of being half-consciously engulfed in the projects they are working on with their hands. These are the mechanics and wood craftsmen who work seven days a week and forget to eat or drink often.

3- THE DUALLY INTELLIGENT: These are the ones capable of incorporating both mental and physical attributes to accomplish any problem placed in their path. These individuals never seem to take a break, rest, or be able to concentrate on nothingness such as meditation. Their mind works allowing the body rest, and the body works allowing the mind a rest. These individuals are the engineers of all industries and professions, the inventors, and creators of artistic works of any medium around them. They are never jobless and are usually the top boss who has earned their position at the top. This group finds it harder than the other groups to stay in one place physically or mentally and are easily distracted, especially if tasked with doing a job they do not like or doing the same job for an extended period. These individuals tend to not stay in one place too long unless bound by life's responsibilities chaining them to their professions.

Playing Out These Traits in Medical Beauty

Innate abilities play a major role in the type and quality of results we as medical practitioners produce. Let's say for example Patricia enters a medical spa facility looking for a particular treatment to rejuvenate and enhance her face for a perceived beauty she has in her mind. Patricia then ventures onto explain, usually not in detail, what she wants to achieve:

The Spatial

The Spatial, from Patricia's verbal description and the Spacial's visual input, can see the problem at hand in a 3-D-like configuration thus visualizing the final result to a point of precision. However, the Spatial may not be able to accomplish this task in totality for Patricia due to a lack of the physical intelligence to manipulate the needle well enough to reach the best target injection site or may not be able to manipulate the needle-cannula (with either filler or thread) easily to travel along a particular course while circumventing the facial tissues (dermal depth, fatty tissue, fascia sheets, muscles, and bone) in the direct path of the needle-cannula to reach a specific target site.

The Physical

The Physical, however, will be able to navigate Patricia's facial tissues with extreme ease to find the perfect target injection sites to accomplish the task. What the Physical may not be able to see is Patricia's true request or what Patricia is really asking for in the way she wants to finally look. Therefore, the Physical may be off target due to a lack of spatial awareness of Patricia's facial feature request. The Physical's ability to accomplish the task to perfection is hindered by the lack of visual geometric points and orientation of the face, especially in real-life animation of Patricia's face.

The Dualist

The Dualist, in this case, can mentally create a 3-D post-treatment picture of Patricia's request and outcome vividly. The Dualist will be able to manipulate, maneuver and navigate with ease to accomplish this specific task seamlessly and without any second guesses of reassurance by Patricia as the procedure is underway. The Dualist, however, has the disadvantage of making errors due to overconfidence and/or a lack of the challenge necessary to thrive for perfection in every case. You see, this is where boredom sets in. These are ADHDs. This is where the Dualist will be working on Patricia's face after gaining insight into what Patricia wants and having the ability to hit the right injection spots, depths, and angles but thinking of the next patient or the last movies seen, or the next thing on their mind. The Dualist cannot always focus every time due to the mundaneness of the task at hand.

The three professional aptitudes described here can render good results every day, all day, if they combine their talent with the skills in good techniques to reach perfection.

Business Owner's Balance: A Force for Change

When someone becomes a business owner, they will be conflicted at the moral and immoral, ethical and unethical, and good and bad decisions they have to make for survival and progression within their chosen field of business. Running a business is similar to being a captain on a ship, and there are many days, weeks, or months that you feel you're not in control depending on what's happening around you. Like running a ship, there is mother nature's constant forces at your back challenging you to fight or retreat.

This is owning and operating a business: everything out there seems like it's focused on destroying what you've created. Your business in some sense has a soul, it's a living functioning entity, but it requires you as the business owner to steer. At times, if the business becomes too big or too challenging for one person to control, it will be incumbent upon the original business owner to hire and delegate duties for sustainability.

The first in charge will be the chief executive officer (CEO) who is responsible for all the stress that you, the business owner, would have otherwise been sentenced to. The CEO is appointed by the Board of Directors but can also be the owner and operator of the company. Most small businesses are owned and operated by the CEO. The CEO is by far the highest-ranking member of a corporation and the highest-paid employee of the corporation. Their job is to direct the managerial staff in the direction of the owner's vision. Therefore, the CEO appointed to the position takes on most of the responsibilities of the owner and is thus paid considerably well and must run that business exceptionally well. Now, since most CEOs are the owners of their companies, they must learn the ropes to excel until they're able to prove a substantial profit niche in that company that they can then sell that company to go on to bigger and better endeavors.

I am in my comfort level as the owner, operator, and practitioner of a small business, and I can tell you firsthand that it is an arduous task to direct and manage your vision for any corporation; yours or someone else's. Though the CEO leaves all the management to the managerial staff, he/she still must manage the managerial staff. As the owner and the CEO of a medical aesthetic spa, many times we are conflicted between the balance of profit and the provision of care.

Some argue that aesthetic medicine deviates from typical medical care since it does not involve curing diseases or alleviating suffering from illnesses. Consequently, the traditional principle of "do no harm" may not apply in the same manner as in standard medical practice. This appealing notion has led many non-medical individuals to venture into opening medical spas. However, when the sense of care and obligation to help others is removed from the practice of medicine, it can become solely profit-driven. Unfortunately, this perspective seems to dominate a significant portion of the U.S. medical landscape, encompassing hospitals, clinics, nursing homes, rehabilitation centers, and various healthcare franchises.

As the owner and CEO, I am responsible for everything that occurs. The purpose of the company and the direction and vision of the company ends with me. The direction of medical care, the implementation of this care and the success of the company is under my direction; however, it is the team of staff working in concert with the CEO that makes any company thrive.

The Responsible Thing to Do is Be Responsible

In the field of medical beauty, there is a difference in how responsibility is assigned compared to standard medicine such as orthopedics, internal medicine, cardiology, obstetrics, geriatrics, etc. In standard medicine, if a patient experiences a negative result, it is common for the blame to be placed on the drug, the disease, or the patient at times, thus shifting the responsibility away from the practitioner. This practice must change for the benefit and welfare of us and our loved ones. However, in medical beauty/medical aesthetics, any negative outcome is visible on the patient's face or body and seen for the world to judge or ridicule; it is solely the fault of the medical provider who performed the injections either by utilizing a poor technique, poor judgment on the required remedy of rejuvenation at the consultation, or by a poor choice of the product—dermal fillers, lasers, thread-lifting needle—to be used on the patient.

So many people have died or suffered from the arrogance of standard medicine, and it is astonishing to me that patients believe and trust every medical provider they encounter whole-heartedly. While I was in orthopedic clinical care and surgery, I witnessed many atrocities that could have been avoided by the treating practitioners whether it was in the hospital or the clinics, and over those 12 years in orthopedics, I was more than determined to carve my own path in medicine and to not do the same as other medical providers I encountered.

Many medical providers have sound knowledge and experience; however, no one would disagree with me that not every medical provider shares the same experience, knowledge, understanding, knowhow, or empathy necessary to be a good provider especially also with the oversight of the insurance conglomerate. I am so proud of the medical practitioners who do not take medical insurance and who stand by their skill, experience, and knowledge in providing care knowing that their success is due to the firsthand results of their patients. They are, at times, called outcasts and mavericks of the industry shunned by mainstream western medicine's fundamentalists.

You see, even if you're not the best medical provider, as long as a medical insurance company covers you, they will send and refer a constant flow of patients every month as long as you follow their protocol in maximizing the benefits of the insurance company. I believe this is where the progression of great care falters and why the U.S. is not the number one medical providing country that it used to be.

Medical practitioners must bear the responsibility of negative outcomes for their patients without blaming the drugs. If the drugs caused the problem, then you must admit that the medical provider prescribed that drug. What if the drug problem occurred with 100 of the medical provider's patients? What's the incentive for the provider to stop promoting or prescribing that particular drug? And therefore, the medical provider cannot blame the drug since there are many measures you can take to see if that drug is compatible with the patient and if it would work well before it is prescribed.

One argument from the medical establishment is that the drug companies make these drugs and therefore, the medical establishments are at the mercy of the drug companies whether the drugs work or not. However, if we force the drug companies to provide the best possible drugs instead of prescribing drugs that are the most well-known or that have a brand name attached to them, patients would fare better.

The Crucial Role of Medical Beauty Experts: Efficacy and Safety in Cosmetic Procedures

Medical Beauty providers, like standard medicine, are entrusted with the efficacy and safety of our implemented treatments. However, unlike standard medicine, efficacy and safety rely predominantly upon us, the medical beauty expert, not just a drug's indication. In standard medicine, drugs are heavily tested, which must meet the Food Drug and Administration's (FDA) requirements to protect the patient's safety. We know that this works most of the time, the intention to keep the public safe is there.

The reality of patients succumbing to their ailments without cures tells us that something is wrong with the end processes of effective drug delivery. In Medical Beauty, hyaluronic acid, bio-stimulators, and dermal threads, the tools we use for rejuvenation, are considered medical devices and not drugs. These medical devices have undergone safety testing and further requirements by the FDA for consumer needs and are deemed safe for use. The actual safety parameters after FDA approval are how the medical beauty provider uses these devices and where on the body they are used.

Some of these medical devices, such as bio-stimulators, if injected in a place on the body or face can lead to devastating outcomes and disfigurement. Therefore, safety relies on proper training and dedication to understanding the limitations of these products despite some marketing tactics to encourage their use. If some of the dermal filler products are injected too deep or too superficially, this can also lead to minor disfigurements and sometimes ulceration and damage to the skin.

All results become technician specific, meaning that the safety, reliability and outcome of your treatment (good or bad) rely predominantly upon who the medical beauty provider is who is injecting your face. Our role as medical beauty injectors become not only the purveyors of these medical devices but the aftermarket approval testers in the reliability of the devices, which leads to off-label treatments of the device and later requesting FDA approval for the areas being tested off label.

In reference to change within the medical cosmetic industry for a better tomorrow with leading-edge drugs and devices geared to safe and effective treatments, big pharma is not the enemy. Big pharma and big equity is just easy to blame. They are the biggest target for our insults, our accusations, and our wrath. However, the real enemy is closer than you think. The real enemy in today's glorified market based on false reporting, fake news, and altered science to set an agenda mostly for profit by you. We have the power to reject inadequate drugs and devices, we have the power of due diligence in gathering information to be informed, we have the power to refuse products from companies not aligned with our values as care providers, we have the power to weed out and report illegal medical services from non-medical perpetrators.

We hold the power to forge positive alliances and ensure that products causing the most iatrogenic illnesses are not perpetuated in the market. It's convenient to criticize and point fingers, only to return to work and inadvertently support the very companies that prioritize profit over well-being. This cognitive disconnect or dissonance permeates the medical professional's world as well. While big pharma and big equity may rightfully earn billions for delivering exceptional drugs and devices, which we, as medical beauty injectors, depend on for our livelihood, there should be no qualms about it. If any of us were to discover, invent, or produce a widely used and beloved medical device or drug, generous rewards would be well-deserved. The discontent often centers on those who resist change and rely solely on faith and hope without taking action to create the necessary improvements.

How Do I Find a Master Injector: Continued Medical Training and Experience is Key

The number of medical beauty injectors is simply astounding and has grown exponentially unlike any other profession we have ever seen. There simply is no precedent for this phenomena, which leaves the government and medical associations baffled at what to do and how to control the rising tidal wave of new injectors from nurses to specialty physicians competing for superiority and dominance. Combing through the search pages of the internet to pick a provider must be daunting and fraught with pure bewilderment. Nothing a practitioner says should be of much significance to your choice, however, what the practitioner does must play a very strong part in your decision-making.

Continued medical education in any specialty or field of medicine from cardiology to medical beauty is paramount to success both for the patient and the provider. Key questions you should be asking to gauge medical beauty provider abilities would be the years of documented experience, which should be posted on their website or adorn the walls, whether medical beauty is the main focus of their career, the approximate number of patients seen daily, and examples of their work via before-and-after pics of previous patients. It is helpful to know that your medical provider is keeping up with the latest technological data and techniques/products for optimal results. These questions are not relegated to only medical beauty, but all aspects of healthcare.

CHAPTER EIGHT

SUMMARY CHAPTER

I covered so much territory in the previous chapters that I felt a summary chapter would help you remember and retain more information. So, here is a brief overview of each chapter.

Chapter One — Enigmatic Origins: Beauty and Aesthetics Unfolded

A Journey into the Visionary Taste of this Island

Caribbean life offers so much more than beautiful beaches during the day and tranquil westward breezes at night. The life of a person in the Caribbean is rich in the distinct island foods, scenic views, and relatively predictable temperate forecasts. The culture here in the Caribbean as I remembered it as a lad was not focused on the consumption or the hoarding of money or wealth for protection of homelessness or poverty, but more on the interpersonal and family relation that governed most conversations. The Caribbean is not fraught with harsh winters, cold days, or humid summers, so island life becomes more of a relaxing journey.

THE LUST FOR MEDICAL BEAUTY

The Beauty of Life in the Islands

Our childhood stresses seem to amount to an enormous amount of grief and anxiety seen from the eyes of a very young and immature adolescent; I was no different.

Determining a Career in this Land of Beauty

Choosing a career as young as 15 years old, in retrospect, is not the very best approach when trying to harness the best abilities of a young lad. The Caribbean has a very laid-back attitude toward work, wealth accumulation, and future planning. This is reflected in many jobs and career choices for the individuals living on these islands. The mode of just making a salary, having a roof over our head and three meals a day is considered success for people with no real-world stresses. It's not a bad life to live; however, it stands in a sharp contrast to the American way of life that's based upon fear. Caribbean life is based upon being chill and relaxing.

Social Status: Opportunities and Resources

The social status of adolescents is defined by the parent's position and role in society based on their education, income, and occupation status (Lareau & Conley, 2008) paraphrased.

Adolescents are the forefathers of their adult selves and play a pivotal role in all activities once out of school. Parents leave their mark that's often buried due to adolescent abandonment of their parents' culture. The normal rebellion of a teenager relates to the death of their childhood and therefore the rebellious nature is that psychological slaughtering of the little girl or little boy within them. Any poor decisions made by that adolescent carry on through the entire 30s 20s and sometimes 40s of their adult life and every dramatic scenario occurring in that child's life is profoundly influential in the type of adult they will become, only held back or tapered by the embedded culture of the parents. The social status of the teenager

146

reflects the social status of one or both of the parents but does not necessarily translate to that influence in the child's adult life and many times that's the opposite of mirroring the parent's influence unless the parents have a pivotal role in the young adult's life.

Sinister Transformations: Beauty Emerges Out of Suffering

Expectations of life at a young age dwindle as you grow older. Expectations of adults with power dwindle as you encounter them and require their assistance for help. We learn quickly from a young age that life is not for the naïve so it's important to look for the bold and strong. The need for help is also governed by the need for assistance and if we receive this assistance at a young age, we're more likely to give this assistance to others as they need us. However, if this assistance at a young age is refused, it's likely that as we grow older, we will refuse the same assistance to anyone looking up to us for help.

Chapter Two — Embracing the Unknown: Leaving the Past and Anticipating the Unforeseen

Growing up is hard to do, some of us could wait until their mid to late 20s, and for the rest of us, high school was the end for adolescence and innocence. My initial impression of the U.S. started with what was advertised on TV and in the pages of foreign magazines, however, having to adapt, meant it had to be done quickly. Every teenager has unrealistic expectations of another country with the allure of starting over from the treacherous teenage life we all know too well.

Journey of Discovery: Finding Beauty Without a Map

Turning 18 years old, with no parental figure, making side hustle money, learning to be street smart, and taking risks with no regard for safety was just another day of my life in Brooklyn, New York. Survival was not a choice, you either did or you did not. Despite the challenges, I made it through high school falling from one frying pan to the other with the bright white light at the end of the tunnel burning steadily. Things looked up but presented additional challenges as I embarked on a volunteer position and found my way to medicine.

Navigating the Judicial System: A Lesson in Inequity

My first encounter with the legal system did not go too well, times were hard, and the city was rough. Blacks and Jews were fighting, Latinos and blacks were fighting, Jews and Latinos were fighting, and the Italians, Irish, Germans, and lower-class whites found a way out of the crosshairs of the English white elites.

Curiosity Didn't Kill the Cat: My Three Saints

My curious nature led me to a new beginning and a path to carving out a life that I felt I deserved. University life was tough, finding permanent shelter was tough, and scraping a meager living together was tougher.

Affirmation: Meeting the Challenges

Graduating from university was a benchmark in my life marking the permanent exit from the life I was thrust into on day one in America. This was a pivotal moment in my life, and I knew I was on the right track and there was nothing that I could not do. Nothing was holding me back besides a marriage that was failing.

The Allure of the Beauty Industry and the Business of Desire

Medicine as a business just did not sit well with me. I stumbled upon many lucrative avenues to turn to, however, the one redeeming step I took was taking a class for cosmetic treatments and facial rejuvenation. With a few training sessions under my belt, I knew this was the path to my freedom from risky medical business dealings that were forced upon us as employees. I was slowly becoming established as a rejuvenation specialist, albeit, in a medical field that was almost non-existent a few years earlier.

Transformations: Evolving Beautifully in Ways Our Parents Could Only Imagine

Our parents didn't have the technology to look better via medical means that were safe and efficient. We have those means today and many of us take advantage of those means and create the external appearance that we would rather present to the world as opposed to presenting the genetic shortcomings of our parents. This was the time to create my professional corporation based on the work I was doing and the necessity to protect my investments, my family, and my income. This was one of the best decisions that I had made along with deciding to invest in myself rather than purchasing property or stocks. that may or may not grow at an average of 10 to 12% per year. The investments in ourselves can be extremely lucrative, thousands of percentages over and above what any other investment would give to you. You just must want it bad enough. And, you must experience loss because it is a powerful catalyst for growth and change.

Chapter Three — Medical Beauty: The History and Emergence of a New World Beauty

Society's demands promote industries. From as far back as early civilization, the necessity to look good and to demonstrate prosperity, made wearing that on your sleeve; you had to prove your status within society by showing others how much more of something you have whether it was goods, spirituality, or physical beauty. As time crawled forward, natural beauty played a significant role in the opportunities for the people who possessed this beauty. Perfect skin was recognized as having a prominent lifestyle with colorful garments that demonstrated the wealth attained. We have not changed that much today; we still recognize and hold to the same values, however with different technologies and materials.

Jennifer's story highlights the difficulties and dangers involved with newer technologies that become more complicated to have, use, and maintain. Introducing elements into a closed system like the human body gives us far more difficulties than just applying products on top of the skin; however, products applied above the skin can also be dangerous but extremely transient. Introducing products within the body can be long-term or forever.

Chapter Four — Vanity's Paradox: Social Pressures to Pursue and Yet Conceal Beauty

This is one of my favorite chapters. The word fame comes from the Latin word VANUS, which means empty inside of something. It relates to an overly positive opinion of one's self and to put their importance and influence above others due to their positive (beautiful) physical appearance.

The word vanity or relating to being vain has become a weaponized word to inflict pain and harm to the individual or individuals spoken about. However, beauty was not always thought of as a negative virtue, it was seen as being pure in heart and spirit. So we heard many stories of beautiful young virgins risking their lives for beauty. Today no one must be considered vain but wish upon themselves all of the positivity that comes with being beautiful.

If I Am Beautiful, Why Do I Need Work Done?

As long as human beings have eyes and use them, we will be judgmental because this sense of vision is linked to our very survival within societies, within civilizations, and out in the wild. Being beautiful is one thing but maintaining beauty is another. Social pressures dictate what we do and don't do. To continue to benefit from the rewards of beauty in society, we must maintain the beauty we have and as that beauty subsides, many will feel the sting of becoming invisible or not cherished as much as when their beauty was prominent and commanding.

Pop culture has played a significant role in the direction of beauty whether it is the face, the body structure, or the clothing we choose to wear. The availability of being presented to millions of people at once as an artist allows that artist or industry's beauty standards to become adopted whether within that country or worldwide.

My 4 S's of Visual Skin Aging

The 4 S's of visual skin aging discuss the primary causes of aging skin. Removing these four dangerous S's from your lifestyle greatly enhances the longevity of your visual presence without the higher cost of medical beauty products and services. Tackling the four S's will also contribute to a natural process just by removing harmful UV radiation of the sun and maintaining the youthfulness and beauty of the skin.

My 4 S's

Sun's UV radiation and its' free radical formations lead to destructive cellular functioning and ultimately diseases along with skin aging.

Stress receptors ignite a barrage of chemical and hormonal changes to the body for protection, however, too much stress will do quite the opposite, causing destructive skin thinning and skin aging.

Sleeping on the face is one of the most destructive habits you can do for your face. Stress lines that are vertical or diagonal will become permanent fissures and create older-looking skin.

Soap is capable of causing superficial chemical burns without you noticing the damage and enough of these burns or a long duration can initiate a complex surface discoloration, rosacea, or dermatitis, which in turn will lead to rapid skin aging.

A Vanishing Act: The Invisibility of Aging

Getting older naturally paves the way for a younger generation to thrive. Unfortunately, that means slowly disappearing or becoming invisible. A younger person will speak to the older generation only if they have to; when we were younger, we did the same. This is why you don't generally find 20-year-olds in close proximity with the older generation, there is not a lot in common and the view of life and what is important is markedly different. Invisibility steps in slowly, and it starts with one or two lines progressing to overall volume loss, height loss and thinning of the frame. This is the natural order of things and should be celebrated rather than feared.

Chapter 5 — History of Aesthetics: Is It Vanity or Simply a Social Need to Belong

History has taught us many things but in relation to beauty, the intentions are the same as a century ago but the tools to achieve external beauty are only now evolving at a pace with the likelihood of transforming medicine as we know it.

Beauty Through the Ages: A Historical Context Exploring Medical Standards

From Barber-Surgeons of the 15th century to the Medical Beauty specialists today, the need for safe beauty transformations is likely to continue in the future.

Traditional Medicine Versus Medical Aesthetics: Exploring Ingenuity Versus Convention

Critical thinking may be a thing of the past when it comes to conventional Western medicine, excessive protocols may be hurting us all imperceptibly, and medical beauty's requirements for optimal results rests in the hands of non-traditionalists.

The Ambiguity of Vanity: Virtue or Vice

Judge not lest ye be judged.

Striking a Healthy Balance

The cost of medical beauty treatments supersedes any other frequent spending on any one service done today. Therefore, the need for discounts and lower rates has put the consumer at a disadvantage, which may be intentional by some. The excitement of a good deal amidst high prices of medical beauty blinds the consumer to promptly trust the injector in hopes of a good result. Unfortunately, you get what you pay for.

The Ethical Practice of Aesthetic Medicine

There is no obligation or mandatory act for any professional to engage in ethical practice, leading to astounding healthcare fraud costs of tens of billions of dollars each year. Healthcare professionals are not gods, and we are subject to immoral actions like any other profession. Trusting blindly is at the patient's peril.

Chapter 6 — Overview of Current Products and Procedures in Aesthetic Medicine

Products Competing for Market Share

Medicine is a for-profit industry.

How Botox Works

The science of Botulinum toxin is revealed in a few easy analogies and explanations. Botulinum toxin does not work on skin wrinkles, but on the nerves which supply an action trigger to the muscles, which in turn are attached to the skin and therefore, the skin benefits.

Not Loyal to a Company, But Loyal to Products

Companies are not people; companies are inanimate concepts. People work for companies, and people are fallible. Products are not fallible, they can't be, and they work or don't work depending on the imperfect people administering them and the parameters in which the products are being administered. If a company has a great product, then the loyalty to that particular company's product that works exceptionally well is defaulted onto the company, and that's just fine.

Not Following the Crowd

Stepping out of the path of the herd can reveal some wonderful pastures not ventured upon yet. Social media has become that well-traveled path leading everyone into an algorithm-guided box of treats for your hard-earned money and attention.

The Science of Fillers

How does anything work? Understanding the science of medical beauty products and the tools used in your rejuvenation journey allows you to make better-informed decisions.

Medical Beauty's Requirements: Knowledge and Understanding.

In my opinion, medical beauty is a fun specialty. Having great results does not have to be an arduous task with awkward moments or uncertainty. It's important to comprehend what is happening to you and why. Learning the fun and exciting ways medical beauty can promote and enhance your appearance gives value to your overall outcome. Know what's being injected in your face and keep a record of the product, the date of the injections, and the practitioner's name, not just the name of the medical spa.

The Side Hustle: Friend or Foe

My foremost obligation in medicine is to the delivery of safe and effective medical care and so it is absolutely imperative to vigorously fight for the availability of better drugs and devices in medical beauty. Along with this guiding principle, championing better medical beauty practitioners goes hand in hand with my values. The decision to venture into other medical specialties as a medical provider is commendable at times but not at the peril of patients. If a practitioner wishes to change specialties or moonlight into other areas, it should be with the same diligence and dedication to the knowledge, procedures, and science of the new specialty.

Personally, I don't want to enter a hospital and be seen by a practitioner who is moonlighting for extra dough. The next time you are seen by a medical practitioner (MD, PA, or NP) make sure you ask to confirm that he/she is practicing their main specialty on you and not their second or third moonlighting gig.

Chapter 7 — Presenting the Diamond Touch Technique

Putting an End to Uncertainty and Madness

This chapter dove into my life work and what is close to my heart. Medical beauty is a craft unlike no other medical specialty dealing with rapid-fire demand from 10-20 people per day wrapped in a blanket of psychological mini dramas where the outcome has to be all about the client. How do you generate nearly 100% patient satisfaction in a minimal allotted time? Only by unwavering commitment to the techniques that reduce drama and elevate peace in the patient as well as the injector.

In my early injecting medical beauty years, anxiety was a major problem due to countless poor results and inadequate patient management. Those days are long gone, enabling me to pursue everything else around this craft for the betterment of it. Creating a technique like no other was a momentous task, but so is re-entering school for your master's or Ph.D. The world needs innovators and self-thinkers, even though many fail and their solutions may fail as well. Innovators are born to innovate and will always rise again.

Negating the Blame

Here speaks volumes of the culture of many professions in the United States. As long as one has a certification or degree, they are considered a professional and as a professional, they know all that is to be known of the topic they are certified for. True learning begins once the schooling stops, and that learning will continue till the death of the individual. As we learn, we undoubtedly make mistakes, otherwise who needs to continue learning? If the mistakes are cast upon the patient or customer, then the catalyst for learning is nullified. Blame, sorrow, defeat, anguish, and guilt are all tokens of blame upon us. Although these negative feelings of blaming ourselves can bring about anxiety and further medical/psychological issues, they must be met with a desire to overcome and squelch the reason for the blame to ensure it does not happen again. Blaming ourselves for our patient's harm is positive for everyone else whom we encounter that requires our help with their medical and psychological health.

The Enthusiast for the Avant-Garde: Starting Over

Starting over your life journey is very hard. Reinventing yourself or finding a side hustle that will lead you to what you truly love as a career is difficult. If you are reading this book and have wondered if you are in the right field, you may think of reinventing your career path and destination. These paragraphs may help you follow a dream of yours in whatever career you choose. Just remember that it is okay to have more than one dream. I have several, and I am doing one of them now. If that side hustle offers a financial resource and you love it, persevere, persevere, persevere. This will lead to your success.

Chapter 8 — Discovering the Perfect Injector

Difference Between a Master of Mind and a Practitioner

The human brain can hold just enough information to do a great job at a few things and never a multitude of things. Someone with a Ph.D. has an immense stockpile of information on just one topic amounting to less than 1% of all information required in this world to survive. This is why there are so many of us. Everyone on this planet is part of a giant organism of different thoughts, and man-ual/psychic abilities, which in a perfect world would lead us all to momentous feats of achievements in every aspect of this universe in a perfect world. In my youth, I often heard the phrase "a jack of all trades and master of none." Well, I still hear this in my head ever so loudly witnessing the number of medical spas creeping up in every neighborhood.

Due Diligence, Trust, and Medical Care

Children do not typically present for medical beauty treatments, adults do. As adults you, and only you, are obligated to do your research on the practitioner who will provide your treatment whether the treatment is part of a medical beauty regiment or standard medicine (from cardiology to podiatry). Medicine is a for-profit business, and so it must be treated that way. Though medical practitioners are dedicated to you and your health, others may not have your best interest in mind when delivering a diagnosis, treatment, advice, or referral.

Medical practitioners are also human beings and subject to fallibility. Unfortunately, there are no great websites (there are a few such as vitals.com and healthgrades.com) to truly have insight into the medical providers available to you other than review sites for medical beauty.

Hopefully, this will change one day if you, the consumer, reach out to the local medical organizations and political representatives for a practitioner review database. Now, verbal recommendations are surprisingly helpful along with Google searches and as always, speaking with as many people as you can about the services of any one particular medical provider and not just a medical spa, clinic, or hospital's published or televised reputation.

Navigating the Beauty Maze: Differentiating Talent

Talent is not just the ability to do something well, talent comes in many different forms, three of which I discuss here regarding the spatial, physical, and dualist forms of talen. I believe everyone has a percentage of these three intelligences from 1% to 99% when it comes to our ability to do something with relative ease as opposed to others. Medical beauty requires them for optimal performance, ease of delivery, and understanding of the patient's concerns and motivations for facial enhancement.

The Responsible Thing to Do is to Be Responsible

This heading has become the common theme of this book, which I am sharing with you. As medical care practitioners, we have a responsibility to the patient first and foremost. If we call ourselves professionals then we need a thorough understanding of not only the disease but also the drugs, the parameters of the causative agents, actions leading to the disease, and the correct advice for sustainable health. All medical practitioners become patients at some time, and I am sure if they do not now share this sentiment with me, they certainly will when their time comes to be treated by a medical professional.

The Crucial Role of Medical Beauty Experts: Efficacy and Safety in Cosmetic Procedures

We are responsible for the fate of our patients who entrust their faces, appearance, and psychological well-being to us. We are the gatekeepers that prevent the less-than-desirable drugs and devices from growing in popularity, which can ultimately hurt millions or billions of people. My one rule of thumb for you the patient/ consumer is that if the drug or device is that good, then everyone will be using it. It will become ubiquitous. Case-in-point, this is true of botulinum toxin and its claims to reduce the appearance of fine lines and wrinkles and it does so remarkably well with very few side effects, virtually no allergic reactions, and if used appropriately, zero deaths. It has great track record. If every drug on the market responded like botulinum toxin, then general health would also be ubiquitous.

How Do I find a Master Injector?: Continued Medical Training and Experience is Key

With the unprecedented growth of medical beauty injectors, many legal gray areas occur leaving attorneys, at times, perplexed on the steps going forward for a liability-free client. Many options are available in the quest for an excellent and experienced injector, however, tried and true is the verbal referral followed by a large online site review platform like Google. Prioritizing the practitioner's actions and history possesses more weight toward a final determination on which medical beauty injector will treat you well rather than the charm or words of the staff. This consideration should be placed across all borders of medical specialties and not just medical beauty.

CLOSING THOUGHTS FROM COLLEAGUES

Introduction from Carl:

Over the years, I have had the privilege of working with and training some amazing medical clinicians in the world of Aesthetic Medicine. As they have been part of my journey to Medical Beauty, I decided to ask them some questions about their association with me and their growth within the industry.

I am truly grateful for the accolades and recognition from my medical injectable experts and peers, as it reinforces the dedication it takes for the love and art of medical beauty. It is an honor to be acknowledged by professionals who understand the intricacies of the field, and it motivates me to continue my pursuit of excellence.

Being able to share my path in this book, *The Lust for Medical Beauty*, is a privilege bestowed upon me that I deeply appreciate. It showcases the trust and respect you all have for the insights and expertise in the medical beauty industry. I am grateful for the opportunity to read your contributions to such an important piece of literature that sheds light on the evolving world of medical beauty and highlights the passion and dedication that drives professionals in this field. Thank you for recognizing my commitment to the art of medical beauty, and I am excited to start the next book diving into the anthropological aspect of human beauty.

Name: Mervat Falah

Credentials: RPA-C
Number of years in industry: 13

Professional association with Carl Clarke:

I have had the privilege of connecting with Carl through his medical beauty WhatsApp group called Cafe Aesthetics hosted and curated by him. I have found the aesthetic chat group to be an invaluable resource for connecting with fellow aesthetic providers and enhancing my practice. Engaging in discussions with other professionals in the field has allowed me to exchange knowledge, seek advice, and gain different perspectives on various aesthetic procedures and treatments.

The group has proven to be an excellent platform for sharing experiences and best practices, particularly when it comes to patient recommendations and addressing aesthetic complications. The collective expertise of the group members has been instrumental in expanding my understanding and refining my approach to delivering optimal outcomes for my patients. I am grateful for the supportive community and the wealth of information this chat group provides, as it has undoubtedly contributed to the growth of its aesthetic providers.

We met personally for the first time at the Injection Anatomy course in New York where Carl is a faculty member. His expertise and commitment to continuous learning and exceptional patient care have made a profound impact on our professional association. From the moment we started collaborating, I recognized Carl's exceptional clinical knowledge and ability to effectively recommend aesthetic procedures and manage aesthetic complications. His analytical thinking and attention to detail have consistently impressed me, allowing the industry to provide comprehensive and accurate care to Patients.

Beyond his clinical acumen, Carl possesses excellent interpersonal skills, making him a valued colleague. His empathetic nature and compassionate approach have fostered strong relationships amongst our colleagues. Carl's ability to actively listen and communicate effectively has greatly contributed to our shared success in delivering high-quality healthcare. His professionalism and dedication to continuous learning serve as an inspiration, as he consistently seeks opportunities to expand his knowledge and stay up-to-date with the latest advancements in our field. Working with Carl has been a truly rewarding experience, and I am grateful for the opportunity to collaborate with such a remarkable physician associate.

The most important thing I have learned from Carl:

One of the most profound lessons I have learned from working alongside Carl is the immense value of professional connections and supporting one another within the medical field. Carl's unwavering commitment to collaboration and fostering a positive work environment has had a transformative effect on my development as a clinician. By witnessing his dedication to building strong relationships with colleagues, I have come to understand that true growth and improvement can be achieved through collective knowledge and support.

Through Carl's mentorship and guidance, I have realized that reaching out to fellow professionals, sharing experiences, and seeking advice not only enhances my clinical skills but also enriches my overall practice. The emphasis on collaboration and learning from one another has expanded my perspective, enabling me to approach patient care with a more comprehensive and well-rounded mindset. Carl's example has ingrained in me the belief that by supporting and uplifting each other, we can collectively strive for excellence and provide the best possible care to our patients. I am incredibly grateful for the invaluable lesson I have learned from Carl Clarke and the significant impact it has had me on my journey as a clinician.

The best part of my chosen profession in medical aesthetics:

Practicing medical aesthetics has been an immensely fulfilling journey for me, driven by the profound impact I have witnessed in the lives of my patients. By helping individuals enhance their appearance and boost their self-esteem, I have had the privilege of enabling them to live their best lives.

Witnessing the transformative power of aesthetic treatments and seeing the newfound confidence and happiness in my patients is incredibly rewarding. It is a privilege to be a part of their journey towards self-acceptance and empowerment. The ability to positively influence their lives by helping them feel more comfortable and confident in their own skin is what fuels my passion for medical aesthetics and continues to inspire me every day.

Story of my best patient outcome:

As an Aesthetic PA, I have had the privilege of helping patients through various stages of their lives. One of my favorite cases, a cancer survivor, came to me seeking to reconstruct her buttock area after undergoing cancer treatment and surgery. She shared with me how the treatment had left her feeling self-conscious and that her body image had taken a hit.

Together, we explored her options and decided that injectable fillers would be the best course of action. The results were beyond what we both expected! Not only did the procedure help to rebuild her lost volume, but it also gave her a new sense of confidence that radiated from within. Watching her light up and embrace her new-found confidence was incredibly rewarding.

Aesthetic procedures are so much more than just physical appearance. It's about helping patients regain their self-esteem and confidence, and it's a privilege to be a part of that journey. My patient's transformation was a testament to the transformative power of Aesthetic procedures. I am honored to have played a part in helping her rebuild her life.

Worst patient outcome:

I once encountered a challenging situation with a patient who had a mental health disorder and struggled to perceive herself as beautiful. Despite my best efforts to provide a satisfactory medical aesthetic outcome, the patient's perception of herself remained unchanged. It was disheartening to witness her persistent negative self-image, as her mental health condition hindered her ability to appreciate any physical enhancements.

This experience served as a poignant reminder of the complex interplay between mental health and body image, emphasizing the importance of a holistic approach to patient care. While the outcome was not what we had hoped for, it underscored the significance of understanding and addressing the underlying psychological factors that can greatly influence the effectiveness of aesthetic interventions.

To skeptical patients:

To a skeptical patient, I understand that medical aesthetics can be a decision surrounded by uncertainties. However, I firmly believe that it offers a remarkable opportunity to preserve your youth and embrace the aging process with grace. Medical aesthetics encompasses a range of procedures and treatments designed to enhance your natural features, address specific concerns, and restore a youthful appearance. These interventions are carefully tailored to meet your unique needs and preferences, with the ultimate goal of helping you look and feel your best. By combining medical expertise, advanced technologies, and artistic techniques, medical aesthetics can effectively target common signs of aging, such as wrinkles, sagging skin, and volume loss. The results are often subtle and natural-looking, allowing you to maintain your individuality while rejuvenating your appearance. Embracing medical aesthetics can empower you to take control of your self-care journey, boost your confidence, and embrace the process of aging gracefully.

Most memorable day in office:

One of the most memorable days I experienced in the office was when I embarked on a unique procedure that had never been performed before. It was an incredibly long and challenging day, requiring significant time and effort to execute successfully. Despite feeling physically exhausted, the immense fulfillment and happiness I felt afterward were indescribable. The sense of accomplishment that accompanied pushing the boundaries of what had been done before and witnessing the positive outcome for the patient was truly gratifying. This particular day served as a testament to the dedication, perseverance, and passion I have for my work, reminding me why I chose to be a part of the medical aesthetics field. It was a powerful reminder that the effort invested in delivering exceptional care and pushing the boundaries of innovation can bring immense fulfillment and joy.

Words of wisdom:

In life, it is crucial to follow your passion with unwavering dedication and integrity. The path towards success is often paved with hard work, perseverance, and sacrifices, but the rewards are worth every ounce of effort. When you pour your heart and soul into your work, it inevitably pays off in ways you may never have imagined. The fulfillment that comes from doing what you love, pursuing your dreams, and making a positive impact is unparalleled. Passion fuels the fire within, propelling you to overcome obstacles, learn from failures, and continually strive for excellence. By approaching your endeavors with integrity, ensuring that your actions align with your values, you build a reputation and legacy that withstands the test of time. Remember, when you combine passion with integrity, success becomes a natural byproduct, bringing immense personal and professional fulfillment along the way.

Name: Durga Sunitha Posina
Credentials: Board Certified MD (Internal Medicine) & Medical Spa Owner & injector
Number of years in the industry: 7

Professional association with Carl Clarke:

I trained with Carl at the beginning of my career in aesthetics. I started training with him on Restylane products, when he began explaining about the product qualities and properties. He had me draw a map of all the products, their G' Primes and categories. Then he went on to explain the anatomy, complications, and demonstrate on our model the different techniques. He started showing us the techniques on the model, then let us do the work and guided us very closely, most importantly if something was not held properly why it's important etc. He also taught his diamond technique, which was very interesting and useful, and most importantly, he then answered all our questions.

The most important thing I have learned from Carl:

The careful organization of teaching materials into layered structures serves to make the effective absorption of knowledge by students easier and more meaningful. Carl used this approach by providing detailed explanations and employing various instructional techniques to enhance the learning experience.

Top two things that impact my ability to practice my profession:

Definitely the complications and the big no no's that he emphasized, and post training I always used to mentally go back to the chart that he made me draw out for reminders and clarification.

The best part of my chosen profession in medical aesthetics:

Every patient is different and carefully chooses what is right for them. My mantra is less is more. I don't believe people should be overusing fillers like a lot of people are, especially encouraging the younger patients to steer away if it is truly not needed.

Story of my best patient outcome:

I had a patient come in who was very depressed because she was losing her hair and she had no idea what to do about it. I used PRP hair restoration with excellent results – she grew back so much hair she was absolutely delighted. This outcome completely changed her life, as prior to this she was depressed to the point of not going out or doing anything with other people because she was so self-conscious about her appearance.

Worst patient outcome:

When I first started injecting Botox, I didn't know how to fix someone who had been to another professional who had done a terrible job and had left them with one eyebrow raised. While I really wanted to help, there did not seem to be a solution to this unique problem.

To skeptical patients:

I would tell them to really do their research and make sure that they find someone who really is a professional and really knows how to apply medical beauty in the best way possible. Good outcomes will truly boost their confidence. However, I would also counsel them to not juggle too many procedures at once; take it easy and tackle one thing at a time.

Most memorable day in the office:

Every day, when I witness each patient walking away with a genuine sense of satisfaction, it fills me with an overwhelming sense of gratitude. Knowing that I, and my colleagues, possess the capacity to bestow happiness and confidence upon someone is an incredible privilege. It's a reminder of the profound impact we can have on people's lives. Whether it's a smile restored, or a health concern addressed, our ability to make a positive difference is a powerful motivator that drives us to provide the best care possible.

Words of wisdom:

Aesthetics is a forever advancing and changing world; always choose a professional who is credentialed, makes you feel comfortable, and most importantly, takes the time to explain and gives their honest opinion of what should be done.

Name: Natalie Eng
Credentials: PA-C
Number of years in the industry: 3½

Professional association with Carl Clarke:

I met Carl at a Galderma training in Boston MA. We automatically became close because we were PAs who work in aesthetics. He was a keynote speaker and presenter. We got to know each other better after the meeting and shared our intel on what it's like to be a PA in aesthetics. He later added me to this WhatsApp group for APPs, who exchange ideas and questions about the industry.

The most important thing I have learned from Carl:

To know your worth as a PA and strive to own your own practice.

Top two things that impact my ability to practice my profession:

In the med spa, I've got a supervising MD keeping an eye on things. I'm all about doing the procedures we have in our lineup. It's not a free-for-all; we stick to the services that are officially on the menu. It is all about safety and quality. It means we're following the rules and making sure our clients get top-notch care. However, it would be great if we could reach a point whereas a professional we can reach a certain level where it is deemed appropriate for us to be a standalone practitioner.

The best part of my chosen profession in medical aesthetics:

This profession has proven to be both enjoyable and financially lucrative. Our work revolves around instilling confidence in our clients, which leads to a consistently contented clientele.

The most rewarding aspect of this career lies in witnessing the transformation of our clients. Observing their newfound self-assurance and the positive impact our services have on their self-esteem is deeply gratifying. It extends beyond mere aesthetic enhancements; it encompasses the elevation of their overall self-worth.

I love that the word-of-mouth endorsements from our satisfied clients contribute significantly to our professional reputation. This, in turn, attracts a continuous influx of new clients eager to experience the benefits of our services. In summary, this profession offers a unique blend of personal fulfillment and financial stability, making it a gratifying and prosperous pursuit.

Story of my best patient outcome:

I enjoy doing Botox and filler on older women (~60s) who have not had any work done. When I show them their reflection in the mirror at the end of a procedure, happy tears fall down their face from seeing their transformation. "I haven't seen myself look like this in years."

Worst patient outcome:

A patient told me he was on the news/TV for work. I injected Dysport into the forehead and he inadvertently got eyelid ptosis, which I reviewed as a possible rare side effect. The side effect lasted about 1.5 months and I kept checking in. The ptosis improved with time and I was able to offer other products that helped during that month.

To skeptical patients:

Do your research, know that patients who ask for a "natural" look, everyone has a different perspective on what natural look or change they want. Know when to stop and listen to your injector when they give a timeline.

Most memorable day in the office:

Currently, there are three pregnant employees in our small office. Two injectors and one receptionist. Watching our patients' expressions as if they are seeing multiple bumps walking around, but in reality, yes, everyone is practically pregnant in this office.

Words of wisdom:

If Medical Beauty is your dream, don't give up! Chasing your dreams means you're diving into the unknown, facing challenges, and learning the ropes as you go. It's not always smooth sailing, but those bumps in the road make you stronger and smarter.

The bottom line is, when your job is your passion, it doesn't feel like a job at all. It's more like an adventure filled with creativity, constant learning, and personal growth.

Name: Merry Thornton
Credentials: Physician Assistant, MBA, owner of Element Medical Aesthetics
Number of years in the industry: 9

Professional association with Carl Clarke:

I met Carl Clarke in November 2020 while I was working at a dermatology practice in Mount Kisco. We had a Galderma filler training with Carl and I remember the first question he asked. "If someone wants their nasolabial folds filled, what do you do?" I had been taught to inject the cheeks and address the upper areas of volume loss first, placing the filler deep, on the periosteum.

While this approach yields beautiful and natural results, it can require a lot of product. Carl went on. "What if they only have the ability to get one syringe? Do you turn them away or do what you can to make them happy?" Obviously the latter. "How do you inject the product and what do you use?" I thought Defyne would make a good choice due to its ability to move naturally with expression. But Carl explained that the high G-prime of Lyft would make it suitable for achieving the best results. I had never thought to inject Lyft superficially, but he showed me various injection techniques in the nasolabial folds and marionette lines to get amazing results that made the patient happy, exceeded their expectations, and would make them want to come back.

Carl told me about a chat group that he moderated with over 100 injectors and added me. It has been an invaluable resource for me over the past three years. Topics in his chat group range from best technique outcomes to legal questions to managing adverse events. I am lucky to be a part of it!

The most important thing I have learned from Carl:

Carl has an entrepreneurial streak and he encouraged me to achieve my dreams of opening a medspa of my own.

Top two things that impact my ability to practice my profession:

1) Visibility as a small business owner. In a world of franchises with big marketing budgets, it can be hard to stand out as a solo practitioner and business owner.

2) As a physician assistant in NY or CT, I need a supervising physician in order to practice. I would like to see this change, as I have been working in this field for almost 10 years and would like to be able to have independence.

The best part of my chosen profession in medical aesthetics:

I love making patients look, and feel, better about themselves. As practitioners, some of our efforts take months to see, and some are immediate. Either way, when the patient sees the improvement, it is a magical moment.

Story of my best patient outcome:

One of my best outcomes was quick, almost immediate, and very satisfying. The patient had gotten under eye filler from another provider a few years ago. She was bothered by her under eye area, which looked puffy and discolored. She assumed this meant she needed more filler. When I told her that the appearance was from migrated filler and that it would look much better after dissolving, she was dubious. After some hyaluronidase, she could not believe how much better the area looked. She was ecstatic, which made me happy!

I also love seeing patients back after getting a full series of Sculptra. They tell me, "my friends say I am aging backwards!" Yet no one can put their finger on what was done because the results are so natural.

Finally, I had a patient who fell down the stairs and had sutures on the chin and below the brow. She was concerned about the scarring. After recommending silicone strips, a topical regimen, and performing RF microneedling with the Genius, her scars are barely perceivable. She is thrilled!

Worst patient outcome:

My worst outcome is when the patient does not see any results, or they are disappointed with the results. This happens less and less with time, as I now know how to manage expectations. If the patient can only get one laser treatment or only get one syringe of filler and I know it will not make a meaningful difference, I make sure to communicate this. The patient can then decide if they want to wait and proceed at a time when they are able to get the full, recommended treatment.

My other worst outcome was on myself! I injected my chin and had a vascular occlusion. But I learned how to manage the situation effectively in case it ever happens again, which hopefully it won't!

To skeptical patients:

The process is a journey. Do not expect overnight results. Take a photo of yourself today and one year from the day you begin your journey. You will see a difference if you stick with me. You have to trust your provider and have open communication. The process takes time because collagen stimulation takes time. Volumization takes time. Improvement of skin tone and texture takes time.

Most memorable day in the office:

The day I opened Element Medical Aesthetics, 3/18/22, was very memorable. It was an exciting time full of eagerness, anticipation, and enthusiasm, but also uncertainty and nervousness! It has been a fun journey and I have learned so much since starting my own practice. Another memorable day came one year later, almost to the day, on 3/27/23. It was my first day back to the office after being out for two weeks for a thoracic discectomy. I was so happy to be back in action with a full schedule and making people feel good about themselves again!

Words of wisdom:

The field of aesthetics is fun and rewarding but also takes time and patience. The consult is the longest part. You have to be an excellent communicator and be willing to have honest conversations with patients. You cannot be afraid to tell someone "no." We take an oath to do no harm, and we must do what is in the patient's best interest. Also, as with any field of medicine, you must keep training and learning to get the best results for your patients.

Name : Yalda Soroush
Credentials: AGACNP-BC, MSN, CANS
Number of years in the industry: 7

Professional association with Carl Clarke:

During the aesthetic training and cadaver courses, I had the opportunity to interact with Mr. Clarke. From my experience, I found him to be a knowledgeable and experienced instructor. He had a wealth of knowledge and expertise in the field of aesthetics, and he was able to communicate this knowledge effectively to the class. He was able to explain complex concepts in a clear and concise manner, and he was always willing to answer questions and provide additional clarification when needed. He was also patient and approachable, creating a positive learning environment where students felt comfortable asking questions and sought feedback.

Throughout the course, Mr. Clarke demonstrated a high level of professionalism and commitment to his work. He was always well-prepared for each session, and he was able to effectively manage his time to ensure that all course objectives were met. Overall, my experience with Mr. Clarke was very positive, and I would highly recommend him to others seeking to further their knowledge and expertise in the field of aesthetics.

The most important thing I have learned from Carl:

By helping me understand rheology and emphasizing the importance of safety, Mr. Clarke helped me become a more knowledgeable and competent practitioner in the field of aesthetics.

Top two things that impact my ability to practice my profession:

As an aesthetic nurse injector and business owner, two things that greatly impact my ability to practice my profession are maintaining current knowledge and skills in the rapidly evolving field of medical aesthetics, and ensuring that all treatments and procedures are performed safely and effectively to meet the needs and expectations of our patients.

The best part of my chosen profession in medical aesthetics:

The best part of my profession in medical aesthetics is the ability to help my patients feel more confident and comfortable in their own skin. It is incredibly rewarding to see the positive impact that aesthetic treatments can have on their self esteem and overall well-being.

Story of my best patient outcome:

One of my most memorable patient outcomes was a woman who came to me with deep wrinkles and sagging skin around her mouth and jawline. Using a combination of injectable fillers and non-surgical skin tightening treatments, we were able to achieve a significant improvement in the appearance of her skin. She was thrilled with the results and felt much more confident and comfortable in her own skin.

Worst patient outcome:

As a healthcare professional, it is important to always prioritize patient safety and take all necessary precautions to minimize the risk of adverse events. While I cannot disclose specific patient information, I can say that any adverse event or poor outcome is always taken very seriously, and we work closely with the patient to address their concerns and ensure their safety and well-being.

To skeptical patients:

I would encourage skeptical patients to do their research and choose a qualified and experienced provider who prioritizes patient safety and has a track record of delivering high-quality results. It is also important to have realistic expectations and to understand that no aesthetic treatment can completely erase the effects of aging or other factors that impact the appearance of the skin.

Most memorable day in the office:

One of my most memorable days in the office was when we hosted a charity event to raise funds for the Autism Speaks Foundation. It was a wonderful opportunity to bring together members of the community and raise awareness about an important cause, while also providing education and demonstrations of our aesthetic treatments.

Words of wisdom:

My advice to anyone interested in pursuing a career in medical aesthetics is to prioritize continuing education and stay up-to-date with the latest advancements and techniques in the field. It is also important to always put the needs and safety of the patient first, and to approach each treatment with care, compassion, and attention to detail.

Limor Oz
Credentials: MSN, APRN FNP-BC
Number of years in the industry: 8½

Professional association with Carl Clarke:

I had met Mr. Clarke in a conference/training Academy for Injection Anatomy presented by Am Spa back in 11/2021. While he was not my direct instructor, he was still extremely helpful and knowledgeable, always very attentive, and always willing to answer any questions.

The most important thing I have learned from Carl:

Every question I asked was always explained in great detail and backed up by science. He always had a specific rationale for every answer, making it very clear and concise.

The best part of my chosen profession in medical aesthetics:

Expressing my Artistry while improving my patient's confidence and looks, through prevention and maintenance as well as applied aesthetics.

Most memorable day in the office:

After a full day of serving clients and having them leave feeling better than when they arrived, I cried because of how blessed I felt because all the hard work was paying off. People trust my knowledge and skills because of all my dedicated work and good results.

Words of wisdom:

I have found that by following my passion and doing what I love, I have been very successful!

Name Christina Sirera
Credentials: RN, BSN - (FNP student)
Number of years in the industry: 17+

Professional association with Carl Clarke:

I met Carl around 10 years ago. He was sent to one of my spas from the company Galderma to show us his techniques with fillers. At that time, he talked about his own Diamond Touch Techniques and was very informative. He even quizzed us after, which I liked because it made me remember what he taught us. He was and is an excellent teacher. Throughout the years, I have had several more training sessions with Carl with Gladerma and I have also had private training with him. I have used him as a trusted contact when I have an issue or need an opinion. He has always responded. He is also the person I have used to do work on my own face.

The most important thing I have learned from Carl:

There are so many. I have loved his technique with Lyft and the building of columns I use frequently, Also, the importance of depth and how you press on the syringe and the rate or speed at which you deploy the filler affects the result. There is a lot more thinking that automatically goes into play when I pick up a syringe because of the training I received from him.

Top two things that impact my ability to practice my profession:

My continuing education in my field is imperative has a major impact on my ability to practice. It is an ever changing field and you have to be on top of the trends and techniques. Also being aware of the ever changing culture is key. Listening carefully to what my clients want is key to delivering the right result.

Best part of my chosen profession in medical aesthetics:

CREATIVITY! Those without the art never get the results that WOW! The art of aesthetics is not taught. The satisfaction of a client that walked in timid and afraid and then leave confident and gleeful. It makes me feel good. It is a selfish "high" I get from creating that feeling in someone else.

BUT, I will say, business smarts is important in this business. This industry is cutthroat and everyone wants in. So many claim to be expert "injectors" and have no idea what they are doing. You have to be protective of yourself and your skills and you have to have a business mind.

Story of my best patient outcome:

I have a client that has had a prior facelift (20+ years ago). She is in her 70s and very thin and also had skin cancer on one side of her face, so the surgery made the face quite asymmetrical. With a combination of treatments including deport, different fillers, and threads she says she looks better than when she had the facelift. She cried when she saw herself. Her friends and family continue to compliment her, and she is more confident and happier than ever. (And so am I!)

Worst patient outcome:

There was a patient that I had treated with fillers and Botox. I thought that she looked great. There was a definitive improvement. She said that she looked horrible and felt distorted and demanded her money back. I said I could dissolve what she didn't like but she refused. She said if we didn't give money back, she would sue. So, she was refunded thousands of dollars, refused to let me dissolve (because in actuality, she liked how she looked) and was able to get a great treatment for free. She tried to come back a year later for more. I declined to treat her. Sometimes you have to "fire" your client.

Another bad outcome was someone who had her eyelid drop after dysport and her daughter's wedding was in three weeks. That was stressful. We prescribed eye drops, even paid for an acupuncturist to help her eye muscle and helped with makeup. The eye still had partial ptosis (drooping but was considerably better.) She is still a client. Sometimes even in the best of hands there is a possibility of an adverse event.

To skeptical patients:

I'd tell them to ask me any and all questions they have. To think about things before they did it and to start slowly. Research your injector. Don't price shop, you get what you pay for. Don't just go by MD, NP, PA, RN and so forth. Look at their reviews, their faces, their office staff. Do they do continuing education in their field? DO they teach? An MD that takes a one-day course is not someone I want doing my injections!

Words of wisdom:

The business side of this industry is almost as important as the education you will need to become a professional injector. In order to have longevity in the field you will need to be aware of the financial business pitfalls you can face. For lack of a better word, each company will try to convince you that their product is best and if you are good, they will use you to "pimp" you out to convince others with your results. Every nurse, doctor, etc., wants to do it "on the side" (that's another type of injector I don't want injecting me. I don't want my face in the hands of someone who does it "on the side"). The "vultures" are the ones who will be so nice to you because they want to learn what you know; learn your skill. Then once they see they can start to make money they will stab you in the back, discredit you and try to steal your business. I have seen and experienced this more than once!

FINAL WORDS OF WISDOM FROM THE AUTHOR TO THE PROFESSIONAL COMMUNITY

1. To ensure a successful career in the business of injectables, it is crucial to master the anatomical face, understand the science of the products you choose, and automate the techniques necessary for both practitioner and patient satisfaction.

2. A healthy work-life balance as a medical beauty expert requires awareness of the potential financial challenges, the impact on both you and the patient's psychological well-being, and the underlying motivation driving your presence in this field.

3. Every company aims for profitability and naturally promotes their products as the best. Understandably, they will want to include you in their goals if you prove your worth. However, it is essential to ensure that the benefits of this partnership are mutually appreciated by both you and the pharmaceutical company.

4. Advocating for and utilizing better products will always lead to a better, more beautiful world.

5. The drive for higher profits can be infectious and may influence certain actions to achieve financial success. Remember to periodically reevaluate your priorities and reconnect with what truly matters to you and your family.

6. Ultimately take your medical oath to its fullest extent to do no physical, financial, or psychological harm.

7. In a field where it seems everyone wants to be a medical beauty injector; your focus should NOT be on competing with others—they will come and go—but rather on challenging and improving yourself. Strive to be the best injector known to man, knowing that this title is transient and intangible.

8. Quality patients seeking quality treatments do NOT want their faces entrusted to someone who views injectables as a mere cash cow, side job, or a "side hustle."

9. Lastly, popularity among the public and your peers as a beauty expert may hold some value, yes, but the true pinnacle of your hard work and dedication lies in the appreciation and meaningful relationships within your own family and personal connections.

Finally, if you have lost the excitement or no longer enjoying what you do then you are missing one of my 3 tenets: ATP (Anatomy, Technique, or Product selection).

ABOUT THE AUTHOR

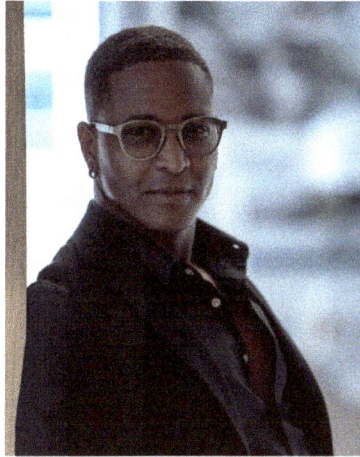

Carl L. Clarke M.H.S, RPAC is a highly accomplished figure in the field of medical aesthetics. With an impressive career span of over 20 years, he has established himself as a leading medical aesthetic trainer, educator, and aesthetic injector coach. Specializing in medical beauty injections, Carl is well-versed in the use of products such as Dysport, Botox, and Daxxify, utilizing these substances to enhance and beautify his clients.

However, what truly sets Carl Clarke apart is his innovative approach to achieving true youthful beauty. Recognizing the importance of slowing down the visual aging process, he incorporates dermal fillers as a modality to enhance one's natural beauty. Additionally, he utilizes dermal threads to offer non-surgical face and body lifts, providing his clients with incredible results without resorting to invasive procedures. His trademarked "Diamond Touch Technique" epitomizes his commitment to delivering low-risk, beautiful outcomes while minimizing the unpleasant side effects such as swelling and bruising.

In addition to his work with clients, Carl is a trailblazer in the industry, having created one of the first internship programs for medical professionals seeking to enter the world of medical beauty. As the owner-operator of Diamond Works Medspa, with locations in both New York City and Florida, he has cultivated an environment that prioritizes consistency and predictability, ensuring both the injector and the patient are wholly satisfied. An accomplished artist and author, he continues to leave a profound impact on the field of medical aesthetics, making him a true influencer in the pursuit of medical beauty.

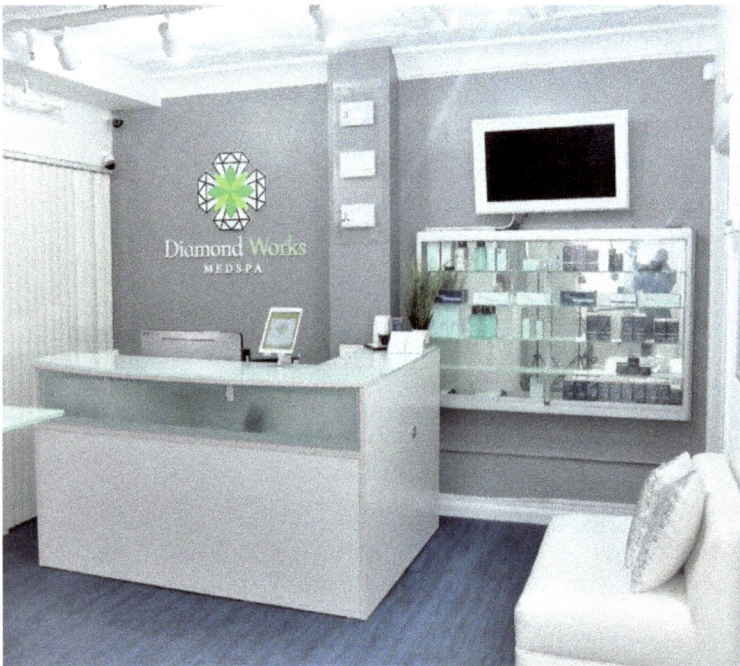

View our results and connect with us on:
www.diamondworksmedspa.com
INSTAGRAM - FACEBOOK - TIKTOK - YOUTUBE
@diamondworksmedspa

www.ingramcontent.com/pod-product-compliance
Lightning Source LLC
Chambersburg PA
CBHW052113030426
42335CB00025B/2963